Slim
Secrets

Slim Secrets

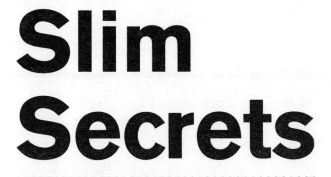

How to eat as much as you like and still lose weight

Anita Bean

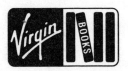

First published in Great Britain in 2008 by
Virgin Books Ltd
Thames Wharf Studios
Rainville Road
London
W6 9HA

ISBN 978 0 7535 1365 1

The Random House Group Limited supports The Forest Stewardship
Council [FSC], the leading international forest certification organisation.
All our titles that are printed on Greenpeace approved FSC certified paper
carry the FSC logo
Our paper procurement policy can be found at
www.rbooks.co.uk/environment

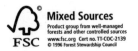

Mixed Sources
Product group from well-managed
forests and other controlled sources
www.fsc.org Cert no. TT-COC-2139
© 1996 Forest Stewardship Council

Typeset by Phoenix Photosetting, Lordswood, Chatham, Kent

Printed and bound in Great Britain by Mackays of Chatham, Chatham, Kent

Contents

Slim
Secrets

Introduction

Are you fed up with diets? They're such hard work – complicated rules to follow, temptations to resist, plans to conform to . . . you try so hard and yet they never quite live up to their promises. Surely there must be an easier way to lose weight?

Well, there is, so keep reading. This book divulges the best-kept secrets of weight loss. Advice that you wish your best friend had told you years ago. It will change the way you eat and allow you, at last, to lose weight (almost) effortlessly (I say almost, because nothing in life comes for free!). You may be a bit sceptical at this point – after all, you have probably read loads of articles on dieting and bought diet books with seductive titles full of empty promises. If you're fed up or disillusioned, I don't blame you.

So how is this book different from all the rest?

- It really works
- It's honest
- It's easy

But it's not a diet. It's a book that teaches you a new – and delicious – way of eating that will help you feel satisfied and full yet allow you to lose weight. It will help you develop a more positive mindset about food and shed old negative beliefs. You'll learn more about how your appetite works and understand what makes you hungry or satisfied. You'll discover how to manage your weight in the long term without feeling hungry all the time. And you'll find out which are the best kinds of exercise you can do.

The advice in this book is proven by science. Everything you'll read is backed by published research. And that's something you don't get with a lot of diet books. The eating system in this book centres on foods that best satisfy your appetite, and foods that give you maximum nutritional benefits for the least calories. The sample 28-day Eating and Activity Plan will help you put the theory into practice, showing you how to eat more for less while losing weight.

What you will read in the pages that follow is the distillation of twenty years of my experience as a nutritionist working with many overweight individuals, including several celebrities. During this time I have listened to their worries, excuses, anguishes and, eventually, joys. I have witnessed the hopelessness they feel, and seen the negative physical and psychological effects that excess weight produces. I have even dieted myself when I used to compete as a (drug-free!) bodybuilder (in this sport, you have to lose as much fat as possible to get that highly defined look – not advisable for the faint-hearted, though). I know from first-hand experience how hard dieting can be. One thing we all have in common is we succeeded in losing weight and keeping it off.

Now you can too. So what are you waiting for?

Enjoy the journey.

Anita

Slim secret no.1
Think Slim

'I'll never be slim,' you sigh, as you open the pages of this book. 'I've tried so many diets but they never seem to do the trick . . . I was born to be fat.'

It's easy to make excuses. It's tempting to blame your genes, your metabolism, your lifestyle, other people, even diets themselves. But at the end of the day you have to face up to the fact: you will only lose weight when you open your mind to the possibility that you *can* lose weight. If you believe you can, you will. If you believe you can't, you probably won't. It's a case of changing your mindset.

In fact, when it comes to losing weight, your mind is the most powerful tool you have. It controls the way you think about food, how you feel about your weight and the way you look. It determines your whole relationship with food. And it is central to your weight-loss journey.

By changing some of your beliefs about food, you can begin to change the way you eat. And lose weight. Where your mind goes your body follows. Need proof? Well, remember when you were learning how to ride your bike? At first, when you wobbled and fell off, you probably felt like giving up. It seemed so hard! But you kept

getting back on, you persisted. You changed your mindset from
'I can't' to 'I can'. And, hey presto! You finally learned how to co-
ordinate balancing and pedalling – you succeeded! If you didn't
believe you could ride a bike, you probably would never have been
able to. That's how powerful your mind is.

Your beliefs and attitudes about your weight can either hold you
back or set you free. The first secret in this book is about thinking
yourself slim – how to change the way you think and take control
of your weight. This will allow you to take the first crucial steps
towards being a slim person.

How did you learn your eating habits?

The biggest clue as to why you are a particular size comes from the
way you were brought up and the way you learned to think and feel
about food. If you can understand how this worked in your family as
you grew up, you'll find it easier to change your eating habits. You'll
also find it easy to pass on positive messages about eating to your
children and ensure they have a healthy attitude towards food.

Did you learn to overeat?

Were you made to finish everything on your plate even when you
were full? Were you forced to eat your greens with the promise of a
sticky pudding?

Most parents worry about their children not eating enough.
Mealtimes are often a battleground as parents coax their children
to eat. But making a child eat when they are genuinely not hungry

overrides their natural inbuilt appetite cues and can cause weight problems later on.

Did you pick up your mother's weight worries?

Was your mother always on a diet or worrying about her weight? Psychologists say that children's attitudes to food and their body image may be passed down from their parents. Children learn by example. If you saw your mother shunning snack foods or counting calories you are likely to do the same. A study at Glasgow University involving a hundred young children concluded that dieting parents, or those who are overanxious about food, may be to blame for their children's unhealthy attitude towards eating and their bodies.

Learn to listen to your body's natural appetite cues

In other words, learn to eat only when you are hungry and stop eating when you are full. Try keeping a food diary, noting down when you are hungry, exactly what you ate and how you felt before and afterwards. This will help you become more aware of your appetite cues and untangle any unhelpful food messages you received as a child.

Don't ban any foods

Try not to attach values of any kind to foods − nothing should be referred to as 'good', 'bad' or 'forbidden'. Don't ban any food − as soon as you restrict a food it becomes more desirable.

Pass on healthy attitudes about food to your children

It may take time to change your negative feelings about food, but in the meantime make sure you don't pass them on to your children. Stop dieting and let your children see that you enjoy healthy food and regular exercise. Share mealtimes as often as possible and eat the same foods.

Don't weigh yourself every day and don't let your children see you on the scales. It's important children learn to eat according to their appetite and enjoy their food, rather than become preoccupied with their weight. Try replacing 'finish your food' with 'eat until you are full' or 'eat as much as you wish'. If they insist on not eating something because they are full, don't allow unhealthy snacks later on. If they are genuinely hungry provide only fruit (or other healthy snacks). Don't ban any foods; just don't have certain items like chocolates and biscuits every day (not having them in the house helps). Allow them on special occasions.

Don't use food as a reward – rewarding good behaviour with sweets only reinforces the idea that they're a special treat and makes children crave them more.

Did your genes make you fat?

Lots of people like to blame their genes when it comes to justifying a bulging waistline. Indeed, fatness often appears to run in families – if you're overweight, chances are one or both of your parents are too. Children with two obese parents have a 70 per cent risk of becoming obese, compared with 20 per cent in children with two lean parents. Studies with identical twins suggest that genes may account for up to 25 per cent of a person's excess weight. Scientists have identified several genes that influence body shape, fat distribution around the body, your appetite (making it larger or smaller), as well as how fast or slow you burn the calories you eat. Genes could even make you prefer fatty food or stop you feeling full when you have eaten.

But diet, activity and other lifestyle habits also 'run in families' – they have nothing to do with genes. These are behaviours children pick up from their parents and carry into adulthood and then pass down to their children. If your family has a habit of eating high-fat food and sitting around, that probably explains the 'family fat'. If, on the other hand, your family is physically active and do lots of sports, you may all be slim and fit.

You cannot change your genes, but you can change your eating and activity habits. Even if the genes are stacked against you, you can be slim – you may have to just eat a little less than others or exercise a bit more.

Whatever your genetic make-up, you still have to eat more calories than you need to put on weight.

In the UK, the number of obese people has doubled in the past twenty years. This, in spite of the fact that we all have the same genes we had twenty years ago. Clearly, it is changes in our behaviour, rather than our genes, that are responsible for making us fat.

Not just genes

Many populations in the world seem prone to obesity. But they only became fat when their natural diet and traditional lifestyle completely changed. For example, the Nauru Polynesians in the South Pacific are the fattest nation in the world, with one in three suffering from diabetes. They became very obese when mining companies moved them off their home island and paid them pensions to sit around all day and eat imported (calorie-dense) food. Their traditional diet of local fish, fruit and vegetables was replaced by a high-fat Western diet of cheap processed meat and refined carbohydrates. Their genes made them especially vulnerable to obesity, but they were not overweight until forced into a couch-potato lifestyle.

Do overweight people have a slow metabolism?

Why is it your slim friend eats what she likes without putting on weight while you only have to look at a cream cake to start piling on the pounds? It's tempting to conclude that she must have a faster metabolism than you. In fact, the opposite is true: the larger you are, the higher your metabolic rate (the amount of energy your body uses at complete rest) will be. This is because, when your body is at complete rest, larger people need more energy to pump the blood around the body and to keep moving. Just as bigger cars use more fuel than small cars, so bigger people use more energy than small people. The hard truth is slim people don't burn up calories any quicker – they just don't consume as many.

What exactly is metabolism?

Metabolism is the term given to all processes by which your body converts food into energy. The *metabolic rate* is the rate at which your body burns calories. Your *basal metabolic rate (BMR)* is the rate at which you burn calories on essential body functions, such as breathing and blood circulation, i.e. when you're doing nothing. It accounts for 60 to 75 per cent of the calories you burn daily.

Why are slim people slim?

Some people seem to have an inborn ability to regulate their calorie intake. They're able to sense when they have had enough to eat and don't overstep the mark. Scientists at Pennsylvania State University in the US call this an inbuilt calorie counter. It's controlled by a gene, which is responsible for giving the brain the message, 'You're full, so stop eating' or 'You need to increase your activity, so exercise more'. That way you don't get fat. A 2003 study at Imperial College, London identified an 'obesity' gene in slim people that protects against obesity. A lot of the time these people think they can get away with eating a lot without gaining weight – but the truth is likely to be that they don't actually eat very much compared to overweight people.

What really causes someone to be overweight?

The hard fact is that if your calorie intake is greater than your calorie output, you will put on weight, as the excess calories from food and drink are stored as fat. If this calorie imbalance occurs for a long time you will end up being overweight. If you eat the same amount of calories as you burn off, your weight will stay the same. But for every excess 7,000 calories you eat, you will gain a kilo in weight.

What is a calorie?

A calorie is the unit used to describe the amount of energy in food. Your calorie needs depend on your age, weight and lifestyle but are roughly 2,000 calories a day for women and 2,500 for men.

Breaking down the barriers

Make a list

Take some time to identify your personal barriers, then write them down. Try to work out exactly what it is that's hindering your progress. For example, at family gatherings you may feel pressurised to eat unhealthy foods or eat larger portions than you would do normally.

Develop your solutions

Now think how you might get past your barriers. Try to think of as many solutions as you can.

Decide on a plan of action

Select one solution you could try. Develop a specific action plan to put your solution into practice.

How to be successful

The reason why some people succeed and others don't has less to do with talent or luck than with how they think. In sport, for example, the difference between the winner and the loser can be very small. It's their mindset that makes the difference.

Small changes in the way you think can trigger big behaviour changes – and successful weight loss.

Take responsibility

Slim people are slim because they take responsibility for what they eat and how they live. They don't need to be told what to do all the time. They decide for themselves how to eat and exercise. You can become slim once you decide to take responsibility for your decisions, which, in turn, will give you greater control over your food intake.

Stop making excuses

'There's nothing I can do about my weight' . . . 'Being overweight runs in my family' . . . 'I have heavy bones' . . . 'It's my genes' . . . 'It's my metabolism' . . . 'It's my age' . . .

Being defensive or blaming your weight on other things won't help your weight-loss efforts. Stop making excuses and trying to justify your weight to others. By continually justifying your weight you are holding on to a negative set of beliefs. Things will never change until you decide to let go of your old attitudes.

Accept yourself

Learning to accept yourself is a good starting point for change. It doesn't mean thinking you are perfect or being complacent about your weight. It simply means being your own friend and accepting that's where you are.

Learn to like yourself

People who dislike themselves tend to punish themselves by doing things they'll regret later on. Guilt sets in and so they punish themselves again, setting up a vicious circle. It goes something like: 'I'm fat, I don't feel good about myself, so I may as well eat more.' So you overeat, feel guilty and even more worthless, and overeat more. The only way to break the vicious circle of overeating is to start liking yourself. Once you feel more comfortable with yourself you'll automatically want to eat healthy food.

Be honest with yourself

If you can learn to be truthful to yourself you will gain greater
control over your eating. How many times have you bought a packet
of chocolate biscuits 'for the children' only to eat them yourself? Or
eaten the leftovers after tea and nibbled your way through supper
preparations without acknowledging the extra calories? Or believed
that snacks 'don't count' if no one sees you eating them. Stop
kidding yourself that you 'hardly eat a thing' and start being more
honest with yourself. Try writing down your food intake – it'll make
you more aware of your eating habits.

Learn from your mistakes

Successful people view their mistakes as opportunities to learn
something from. When you fell off your bike, you worked out what
you did wrong and learned how to get it right next time. You didn't
give up – you kept trying until you succeeded. Next time you eat
a few biscuits too many, don't beat yourself up about it. Learn
something useful from the circumstances surrounding your mistakes
and decide how you will deal with the situation next time. Just say,
'OK, that's what I did this time – what will I do differently next time?'

Focus

Successful people are totally focused. The goal they are focused
on is their own rather than someone else's. They aren't following
someone else's dream, or diet plan, or exercise programme. If you
want to be slim, you have to focus on this goal 100 per cent. The

reason you haven't succeeded up to now is that you haven't been focused on it properly. Chances are you focused more on being overweight and how miserable it made you feel. It's like making a shopping list of things you don't need. It would take you an awful long time to get your shopping done as you'd be distracted by all the things you'd decided not to buy.

Decide to take control

Does your weight control you or do you control your weight?

It's tough to face up to it but you need to take sole responsibility for your weight. If you don't, then no one else will! You can choose to change your weight. You have the power to control your weight – not the other way round. By taking more control of your eating you take more control of your life in general.

Start believing in yourself

If you believe you can't change your weight, you'll stay the way you are. You have to believe that you *can* control your weight and that you *can* be healthy and slim. If you hang on to the same old beliefs, your eating habits won't ever change, nor will your weight. You won't be in control.

Change your mindset

Once you change your mindset and start thinking like a slim person (even if you're not one yet) you'll change your relationship with food and your eating habits. You'll automatically make healthier food choices.

Build self-esteem

If you have a poor self-image, food is more likely to be controlling you rather than you controlling your food intake. Psychologists believe people who are unhappy and don't really like themselves are more likely to have a weight issue. But losing weight itself won't boost your self-esteem – it's the other way round. To lose weight, first you need to start liking yourself and take control of your life. Only by regaining control will you stop feeling helpless about your weight. In turn, this will boost your self-esteem and you'll be able to tackle your weight problem.

You don't have to seek approval from others

People who constantly seek approval from others have low self-esteem. Teach yourself not to worry about what other people think of you.

Assert yourself

Don't be afraid to assert yourself when you don't want to eat something just because everyone else is eating. Learn to say 'no, thank you' when other people push you to eat or when you are full.

Are overweight people less happy?

People who are happy within themselves and like themselves tend to be at a healthy weight or at least a weight that they are genuinely happy with. People who have a tendency to be overweight are more likely to be unhappy with themselves and lack self-esteem. They often have a negative self-image, believing they don't have the ability to do anything about the things they are unhappy with, such as their appearance.

Happiness, self-esteem and weight are very much intertwined. If you don't like the way you look, you tend to feel negative about yourself and have low self-esteem. This leads to feelings of helplessness and feeling powerless about your weight, so you eat more and exercise less. Thus a vicious circle sets up.

How to think like a slim person

Slim people are slim because they have chosen to be slim. They have accepted responsibility for their weight and they control it through their eating and exercise habits. By changing your old set of beliefs, you too can begin to think like a slim person.

Get organised

If you feel out of control in other areas of your life, this can add to low self-esteem and out-of-control eating. Even if your day has to revolve around the kids or your boss dictates your workload, you can gain a greater sense of control just by being more organised. Start by clearing out cupboards, tackle overdue paperwork and keep a diary to manage your time better.

Take time to change

Don't expect instant results after making a change. A lot of people are disappointed when the scales register only a modest change in their weight after a week's dieting. All that hard work for such a small benefit, you may think. But it may take a while, maybe even a few weeks, to really reap the benefits. After all, it took you a long time to become overweight, so give yourself a realistic amount of time to reverse the process.

Stop feeling deprived

If you keep thinking you're deprived or missing out, you'll never succeed in losing weight. Once negative thoughts creep in they can drag you back and keep you enslaved to your old (unhealthy) eating behaviour. You need to talk yourself into a positive attitude, and stop feeling sorry for yourself. Talk to yourself in a way that's motivating when your inner dialogue rears its ugly head.

Have a strategy

Weight loss is not about willpower. Those who succeed at weight loss do not have greater willpower than those who fail – they just have better strategies.

Write it down

One thing is clear from the hundreds of studies on weight loss. People who write down what they eat each day lose more weight and are better at keeping it off than those who don't. So write down everything you eat. Keeping a food diary will give you a much clearer idea of where your calories are coming from. Write down everything you eat and drink for one week (or longer if you can manage it), noting the portion weights and sizes. Try to be as accurate as possible, recording the weights of everything and remembering to write down every snack and every drink. Be as honest as possible – that handful of crisps, those biscuits while making tea, that glass of wine after work. You may be surprised how quickly the calories add up or how often you nibble.

Look at your food diary and identify the foods or drinks that really aren't helping your fat-loss efforts. Work out which types of food you need to reduce or increase. The main culprits are likely to be calorie-dense low-fibre snacks: biscuits, puddings, crisps, ice cream, cakes and chocolate bars.

Identify the triggers

Work out which foods cause you to overeat – the ones that you find almost impossible to resist. Keep these problem foods out of your home. If it's not there, you won't think about it as much and be tempted to overeat.

Eat regular meals

If you eat chaotically, you lose the ability to make the connection between hunger and eating – and the result is overeating. Developing a predictable and stable meal pattern is crucial. The reason most diets work initially is because they give your eating habits structure, usually three meals a day and maybe a healthy snack. This helps to rein in out-of-control eating. But often dieters become fixated with some other diet rule (such as calories or carbohydrate units) and alter the structure of their eating habits, skipping breakfast or delaying lunch, for example. And that's when the diet starts to go wrong. Plan to eat three meals a day plus two small, healthy snacks.

Never undereat

Don't skip meals or snacks. Depriving yourself can lead to overeating later on. When you let yourself get really hungry it's harder to make slim choices. You're more likely to give in to temptation as you pass the baker's shop or grab a chocolate bar on the run. Or you can convince yourself that you need extra food to satisfy your hunger. Plan what and when you will eat and avoid long gaps between meals. Take a healthy snack with you so you won't have to eat whatever is to hand.

Follow the 80/20 rule

The key to long-term success is balance and moderation. So follow the 80/20 rule. It's what you do *most* of the time – i.e. 80 per cent – that counts.

Don't deny forbidden foods

Consistently denying yourself a forbidden treat isn't the way to lose weight at all. It tends to set up a psychological state of deprivation, and once that abstinence is broken, you enter a state of rebellion, which can lead to eating every scrap of food you can get your hands on. If you always restrict what you eat you are more likely to lose control and overindulge when you taste the forbidden food. Allow yourself to eat what you want, but decide beforehand how much you are going to have – and stick to it!

Compensate

A slim person automatically compensates for overeating. If they overeat one day they just get back on track the next day. Get into the habit of listening to and acting on the body's hunger cues (e.g. you won't feel as hungry after a big meal). If you've overindulged, eat a little less at your next meal or the next day or take a bit more exercise. It's called calorie balance: making sure your calorie intake equals your calorie output.

Diets don't work long term

Diets don't lead to lasting weight loss for the majority of people. In 2007 researchers at the University of California reviewed 31 previous studies and found that during the first 6 months of a diet people typically lost between 5 and 10 per

> cent of their weight, but within 5 years two-thirds of people put more weight on than they had lost. Most would have been better off not going on the diet at all.

How to change your mindset

It's easy to defeat yourself with self-sabotaging beliefs without even being aware of them. Your beliefs and attitudes condition you to expect certain outcomes. They shape your behaviour and mould your habits. They set you up to succeed or fail. To succeed on your weight-loss journey you need to change some of your old beliefs that may be keeping you overweight. Here are some of the most common ones – and how to change them.

Old attitude

I'm desperate to lose weight but I'm afraid, however hard I try, I won't succeed.

New attitude

I can be slim if I want to.

If you believe you can't lose weight then it will be a self-fulfilling prophecy. You can lose weight if you want to by changing negative thoughts into positive ones. Reprogramme yourself for the results you want by thinking like a slim person and believe that you were meant to be slim. Try saying, 'I am a naturally slim person. I will lose

weight by choosing nutritious foods that are good for my body.'
Return to these thoughts every day and soon they will become part
of the new positive way you think about yourself.

Old attitude

**Losing weight means giving up all my favourite foods. Life
wouldn't be worth living!**

New attitude

**I can still eat my favourite foods but I just need to set limits
for how much.**

Banning favourite foods is not the answer. As soon as a food
is deemed off-limits you start thinking about it all the time and
crave it until you finally give in to temptation and overeat. Allow
yourself that food at specified times or designated days. For
example, if it's chocolate you crave, break off a couple of squares.
Then eat them slowly, don't scoff them. Enjoy every mouthful. The
chances are you'll feel more satisfied than if you had eaten the
entire bar. The rest of the time, keep tempting foods out of sight at
home.

Old attitude

**I don't have time to lose weight – it takes too much
effort.**

New attitude

I'm going to make weight loss a priority and focus on preparing healthy food and taking a bit more exercise.

Lack of time is probably the most common excuse. But you don't need extra time to make weight loss work for you. It's a case of prioritising your goals, planning your meals and snacks so you always have healthy foods to hand, and making simple changes to the way you shop and how you cook.

Old attitude

I can't lose weight because I'll feel hungry and weak.

New attitude

I will focus on eating plenty of healthy foods that satisfy my hunger. If I get hungry then I'll eat a healthy snack.

In Chapter 2 you will learn which foods satisfy your appetite best. And in Chapter 3 you'll discover which foods have the greatest filling power for fewest calories. Including these foods in your diet will help keep hunger pangs at bay.

Old attitude

I have a social occasion coming up so there's no point trying to lose weight.

New attitude

I will develop some good strategies to help me cope with tricky times.

Social occasions are no excuse for why you can't eat healthily. No one forces you to overeat – you can choose what you eat! Pick the healthiest dishes – have larger portions of low-calorie foods and only small portions of treats. At buffets, put food on your plate then move away from the food table, and select only a few different types of foods. Don't feel you must eat everything on offer, avoid second helpings (learn to say 'no'), and when your taste buds are satisfied stop eating.

Old attitude

Every time I lose weight, it just goes back on again, so I might as well not bother.

New attitude

Healthy eating is something I want to stick to for a lifetime.

Most diets are restrictive and cannot be kept up for long because they require too many drastic changes. The solution is to make gradual changes to your eating habits that you know you can stick to. Avoid quick-fix diets – they don't retrain long-term eating habits.

Old attitude

I'd like to lose weight but I haven't got enough willpower.

New attitude

I will make a list of the reasons why I want to lose weight and set myself a good goal.

If you know there are good reasons for what you're doing you'll find it easier to stay the course. If you write down your goals you're more likely to achieve them (see 'How to set your goals' next). Read through your list every day to help you keep focused. Practise visualisation and start to believe that your goal is possible.

Old attitude

There's no point trying to lose weight. Even if I hardly eat a thing my weight doesn't change.

New attitude

Weight loss may be harder for me than other people but I can still do it if I'm honest about what I eat.

Many dieters eat more than they think they do. A US study found that women typically reported eating 400 fewer calories than they actually ate. Try measuring your food and keeping a food diary to see exactly what you eat and where your downfalls lie.

Choose smaller portions of calorie-dense foods (desserts, cheese, margarine) and fill up with foods that have a low-calorie density (fruit, vegetables, salad). See chapter 3 for more details on this.

How to set your goals

Research has shown that people who set good goals are more likely to be successful in making changes. In a study at City University, New York, where participants had to try to increase their fibre intake, the intake of the groups that had set specific goals was nearly double that of the other groups.

It may sound obvious, but goals help focus your mind. They help to keep you on track. Not having a goal means allowing circumstances or other people to determine your fate. The first step is to assess where you are now and where you want to be. Then write it down in as much detail as possible. A good goal is made up of five elements:

S	=	specific
M	=	measurable
A	=	agreed
R	=	realistic
T	=	time scaled

Let's look at these SMART elements more closely.

Specific

Your long-term goal can be broad in scope, but your short-term goals must be quite specific. That means stating a clear aim of what you want to do. Avoid vague statements about what you hope to achieve. So, instead of 'I want to be slim' write 'I want to wear size 12 jeans'.

Your goals also need to be personal – research shows that it is the internal motivators that really drive people to success – so write down the reasons why you want to lose weight and how losing weight will improve your life.

Measurable

You need to be able to measure your progress, otherwise you won't know whether you have reached your goal. So state your goals in terms of weight loss, clothes size, body-fat measurements, or body-circumference measurements. Keep a record of your progress and evaluate your goals once a week to see if you are staying on target.

Agreed

Commit your goal to paper – this signals a commitment to change. You will be much more likely to achieve your goal than if you simply kept it as a thought in your head. Write it in the form of a personal mission statement; then sign and date what you have written. Place a copy somewhere you can see it each day, such as on your desk, a bulletin board or on the fridge. That piece of paper will constantly remind you that your goals are waiting to be achieved. Aim to read your goals every day. Like a legal contract, this technique will keep your mind focused.

Realistic

Your goal should be realistic – attainable for your body size, natural shape and lifestyle. There's nothing wrong with aiming for the top but, at the same time, be realistic. It's OK to push yourself but you must also look objectively at yourself when deciding if the goal is realistic. On the other hand, don't set a goal that's too easy to attain – otherwise you won't be motivated to achieve it. For example, aiming to achieve a hip measurement of 34 inches (85cm) may be unrealistic for your natural frame. Instead, choose a favourable measurement that you have been in the past and aim to achieve that within a realistic timescale. When setting a weight-loss goal, bear in mind health professionals recommend a weight loss of half a pound to a pound (¼–½kg) per week. You're more likely to sustain this loss over time.

Time scaled

Now you need to set a clear and realistic timescale. Decide on a deadline – this prompts action and will help set your plan in motion. Without a clear timescale, it's easy to put off starting your programme and you'll end up never achieving your goals.

It is also helpful to break up your goal into distinct segments, as this helps you focus on the progress you make each week. For example, if your major goal is to lose two stone (28lb) break it down into smaller goals of, say, seven pounds spread out over the course of four months, and then weekly goals of one to two pounds. When you have reached your first mini-goal move on to your second target. Rather like climbing the rungs of a ladder, focus on one step at a time. Each step moves you closer and closer to the top – every pound you lose is a step nearer your target weight loss.

Reward yourself

Rewards can help you stay enthusiastic. Give yourself rewards when you have reached a goal, no matter how small. This could be something as simple as a star or smiley face on your calendar, a relaxing bath, or allowing yourself time to read the entire Sunday papers for reaching your weekly target. For reaching the bigger goals decide on a special treat like a beauty treatment, new make-up, a trip to the theatre, new clothes, or a new CD. Or you could put aside a little money each time you reach a small goal then treat yourself to something when you reach a bigger goal. Try to focus on rewards that are not food related but still bring you enjoyment. Make a list of some small and big rewards you can look forward to.

Should I carry on wearing my old baggy clothes as a constant reminder that I need to lose weight?

Definitely not. Wearing baggy clothes makes people feel unattractive, so will demotivate rather than motivate you to lose weight. I recommend that you treat yourself to some new clothes when you start to lose weight – and continue doing so. Not only will you feel slimmer and more confident but, also, having clothes that fit will help you notice any changes more easily, which is a further motivator as you continue losing weight. Don't put off buying new clothes until you reach your goal weight or size. This is like putting your life on hold until you become slim — you're more likely to feel frustrated if you don't see results quickly. Buying new clothes, even if you wear them for only a short time, is an investment in your weight-loss journey. It will boost your self-esteem and serve as an incentive to stick to your plan. It's also a commitment — once you've spent extra money on clothes you are more likely to continue making an effort to adopt new healthy-eating and activity habits. Don't make the mistake of buying clothes that are too small, i.e. the size you *want* to be, as you can't predict exactly what shape you'll be in the future. Wearing clothes that fit, on the other hand, will make you look and feel better and remind you of your progress, not how far you still have to go.

How to visualise success

Visualisation is a great way of motivating and speeding you towards your goal. It's used by sportspeople to help them focus on their performance and banish negative thoughts. It's simple yet extremely effective. Have a clear mental picture of how you will look when you achieve your goal. Make it three-dimensional and use as many senses as possible to bring that image to life. Imagine exactly what you'll look like and what you will be wearing. Now imagine how you will feel when you achieve your goal. Will you be feeling satisfied and happy? Cool and in control? Excited, loved, interested, glamorous, confident? Imagine what you would hear. You might hear people paying you compliments or you may hear a voice in your head telling you how great you look. Imagine other sounds around you, such as music, to help bring that image to life. Try putting it all together and make a film in your mind of the new slim you. Give it a soundtrack. Make yourself the star. Keep replaying that film over and over. Soon you'll make it a reality.

How to keep on track

Monitor your progress on a regular basis so you can check that your actions are producing the results you want. If they are not, you need to take the necessary steps to get you back on track. Keeping a daily food-and-activity diary or weekly weight chart can be great motivators. Look back over your notes at the end of each week. If your achievement matches your goal, reward yourself. Don't use weight as the only measure of your progress, otherwise it's very easy to give up if the scales aren't telling you what you want them to. It may take a while for your weight to reflect all the changes you make. It may be useful to record the following details:

- What and how much you ate each day
- Details of the activity and exercise you took
- Your body measurements, such as percentage body fat, waist, chest, hip, leg and arm circumference measurements, or just how snugly your clothes fit
- Changes in your mood
- Changes in your sense of wellbeing and self-esteem

Photographs taken before you start your new programme and then at intervals throughout your training will help to give you feedback on your progress. This is more objective than simply looking in the mirror.

Get support

Get as many of your friends and family as possible to support you in your efforts to lose weight. Let them know the details of your plan and how they can help. This may include helping you plan menus, prepare meals, or joining you for a walk, gym visit or other activities. They can help ensure you stick to your eating and activity programmes. They should be able to motivate you when the going gets tough. In fact, they may even want join you! See if you can team up with a friend or partner — someone who is also interested in losing weight. You can give each other lots of encouragement, listen to each other and help each other get over the rough spots. This kind of supportive relationship will strengthen your commitment and make your journey more enjoyable.

Don't let anyone discourage you from your plans — stay away from negative and unsupportive people who are sceptical of your new plans. Some people may try to undermine your efforts, so don't discuss your plans with them.

Get a mentor

Consider asking someone whose achievements you respect to mentor you. This often works best with someone outside your immediate circle of family and friends. A partner or close friend may not be the ideal person to offer unbiased advice or constructive criticism.

Are you the right weight for your height?

Use this BMI chart to calculate your body mass index. The theory behind this chart, which is used in obesity research, is a mathematical formula called the Body Mass Index (BMI). The BMI is calculated by dividing your weight (in kilos) by the square of your height (in metres). For example, if your weight is 60kg and height 1.7m, your BMI is 21:

$$60 \div (1.7 \times 1.7) = 20.75$$

If your BMI is between 18.5 and 24.9, this is healthy. Your goal should be to maintain your weight at this level. Between 25 and 29.9 is overweight, while a BMI of 30 or more is defined as obese.

As most people in the UK still measure their height in feet and inches and their weight in stones and pounds, the table here gives Imperial values for convenience. To use the table, select your height then select your weight (select the nearest value/s to your own if they are not displayed in the chart). Your Body Mass Index will be listed at the top and bottom of the BMI chart.

BMI	19	20	21	22	23	24	25	26	27	28	29	30	31	32	33	34	35
Height (inches)	Body Weight (stone)																
58" (4'10")	6.5	6.9	7.1	7.5	7.9	8.2	8.5	8.9	9.2	9.6	9.9	10.2	10.6	10.9	11.3	11.6	12.0
59" (4'11")	6.7	7.1	7.4	7.8	8.1	8.5	8.9	9.1	9.5	9.9	10.2	10.6	10.9	11.2	11.6	12.0	12.3
60" (5')	6.9	7.3	107	7.6	8.4	8.8	9.1	9.5	9.9	10.2	10.6	10.9	11.3	11.6	12.0	12.4	12.8
61" (5'1")	7.1	7.6	7.9	8.3	8.7	9.1	9.4	9.8	10.2	10.6	10.9	11.3	11.7	12.1	12.4	12.9	13.2
62" (5'2")	7.4	7.8	8.2	8.6	9.0	9.4	9.7	10.1	10.5	10.9	11.3	11.6	12.1	12.5	12.9	13.3	13.6
63" (5'3")	7.6	8.1	8.4	8.9	9.3	9.6	10.1	10.4	10.9	11.3	11.6	12.1	12.5	12.9	13.3	13.6	14.1
64" (5'4")	7.9	8.3	8.7	9.1	9.6	10.0	10.4	10.8	11.2	11.6	12.1	12.4	12.9	13.3	13.7	14.1	14.6
65" (5'5")	8.1	8.6	9.0	9.4	9.9	10.3	10.7	11.1	11.6	12.0	12.4	12.9	13.3	13.7	14.1	14.6	15.0
66" (5'6")	8.4	8.9	9.3	9.7	10.1	10.6	11.1	11.5	11.9	12.4	12.8	13.3	13.7	14.1	14.6	15	15.4
67" (5'7")	8.6	9.1	9.6	10.0	10.4	10.9	11.4	11.9	12.3	12.7	13.2	13.6	14.1	14.6	15.1	15.5	15.9
68" (5'8")	8.9	9.4	9.9	10.3	10.8	11.3	11.7	12.2	12.6	13.1	13.6	14.1	14.5	15.0	15.4	15.9	16.4
69" (5'9")	9.1	9.6	10.1	10.6	11.1	11.6	12.1	12.6	13.0	13.5	14.0	14.5	14.9	15.4	15.9	16.4	16.9
70" (5'10")	9.4	9.9	10.4	10.9	11.4	11.9	12.4	12.9	13.4	13.9	14.4	14.9	15.4	15.9	16.4	16.9	17.4
71" (5'11")	9.7	10.2	10.7	11.2	11.8	12.3	12.8	13.3	13.8	14.3	14.9	15.4	15.9	16.4	16.9	17.4	17.9
72" (6')	10.0	10.5	11.0	11.6	12.1	12.6	13.1	13.6	14.2	14.7	15.2	15.8	16.3	16.8	17.3	17.9	18.4
73" (6'1")	10.3	10.8	11.4	11.9	12.4	13.0	13.5	14.1	14.6	15.1	15.6	16.2	16.8	17.3	17.9	18.4	18.9
74" (6'2")	10.6	11.1	11.4	12.2	12.8	13.3	13.9	14.4	15.0	15.6	16.1	16.6	17.2	17.8	18.3	18.9	19.4
75" (6'3")	10.9	11.4	12.0	12.6	13.1	13.7	14.3	14.9	15.4	16.0	16.6	17.1	17.7	18.3	18.9	19.4	19.9
76" (6'4")	11.1	11.7	12.3	12.9	13.5	14.1	14.6	15.2	15.8	16.4	17.0	17.6	18.1	18.8	19.4	19.9	20.5
BMI	19	20	21	22	23	24	25	26	27	28	29	30	31	32	33	34	35

The BMI is a useful method but it doesn't take into account where fat is stored in your body. This is important because so-called apple-shaped people (with most of their fat stored around the abdomen) are more at risk of developing obesity-related diseases such as type 2 diabetes, high blood pressure and heart disease, than pear-shaped people who have most fat on their hips. The BMI also does not allow for how much muscle you have. Try the following tests to find out your health risk:

Apple vs. Pear

To assess whether you are an apple or a pear, divide your waist measurement by your hip measurement: if the figure is greater than 0.85 for women or 0.95 for men, you are an apple and more at risk from diseases linked to obesity.

Waist circumference

Many experts now favour waist measurement as a better indication of whether or not you are overweight. It reflects the amount of fat you carry in your abdomen and is regarded as more accurate than BMI in predicting type 2 diabetes risk. If a woman's waist measures more than 34 inches (88cm) and a man's more than 40 inches (102cm) then they need to lose weight.

Slim secret no. 2
Satisfy Your Hunger

Sarah is 43 years old and has attempted to lose weight many times over the years but somehow never manages to keep it off. She generally looks after her body well, she goes to the gym at least twice a week, her diet is fairly healthy, but all her past weight-loss attempts have resulted in the same predicament: she is hungry all the time. 'Throughout the day, I feel I want to snack even after I've just eaten. I spend most of my time thinking about food, planning what I'll eat at my next meal. Eventually, I just give in to my hunger and eat anything to hand. I end up putting back the weight I've lost.'

If you recognise what Sarah is experiencing, you're not alone. The reason diets often fail is simple — they don't satisfy your hunger. They require you to eat smaller portions than usual in order to eat fewer calories. But the problem with eating less food is that you end up feeling hungry and deprived. Small portions simply don't fill you up or satisfy your hunger. That's why most diets are not sustainable. Sooner or later you'll give in and overeat.

In this chapter, you'll learn about the science of appetite and why you get hungry (psychological and emotional hunger are explored in Chapter 5). You'll learn about satiety, the feeling of satisfaction after eating a meal, and which foods you should eat to stave off hunger.

You'll soon develop a greater ability to listen to your body's natural hunger cues, curb your appetite and stop overeating. In short, you'll gain greater control over your food intake.

What's the difference between hunger and appetite?

Sometimes it's hard to know whether you're really hungry or whether it's just your head urging you to eat more than is good for you. Is it your appetite or is your body in need of fuel? The two are, in fact, quite different. **Hunger** is that disagreeable feeling caused by the need for food. **Appetite** is your desire for food, a pleasant sensation felt in anticipation of eating. Knowing more about the way your appetite works can make the difference between you controlling your eating or it controlling you.

How your appetite works

As a baby you had no problem knowing when you were hungry and when you were full. Your appetite-control mechanism worked perfectly, balancing your intake with your needs. But very early in life you learned how to override your natural hunger signals and it became easier to overeat. Studies show that when young children are presented with a large portion they will eat all of it in spite of feeling full.

Scientists have learned a lot in the last few years about what controls appetite. There's still some way to go but one thing is clear: your urge to eat — whether you're truly hungry or not — is a complex interaction between your psychology, your biology and your surroundings, masterminded by the hypothalamus in your brain.

Your brain receives hunger signals from your gut and your bloodstream (which tell your brain to eat), satiety signals from your gut and your fat cells (which tell your brain that you are full or need to stop eating) and 'emotional messages' from another region of the brain called the cortex, which can override true hunger messages so that even if your body says it's not hungry, your emotions can signal your brain that it's time to eat. The whole process involves more than twenty different hormones or chemical messengers.

The hunger-off switches

The satiety centre in your brain receives short-term signals from the gut and long-term signals from your fat cells. Satiety is that pleasant feeling of fullness and satisfaction you get during and after eating a meal.

Short-term signals

Within minutes of starting eating, stretch and chemical receptors in your stomach lining signal to the brain that you have eaten something. Cells lining your intestines then begin to release chemical messengers – cholecystokinin (CCK) and glucagon-like peptide 1 (GLP-1) – as you carry on eating. These highly potent appetite inhibitors tell the brain to stop eating. However, it takes around twenty minutes after beginning a meal for this signal to get through. So if you scoff your food in, say, ten minutes, you will almost certainly overeat before your brain receives the full-up messages from your gut. A study at the University of Florida found that people eat up to 15 per cent more calories when they rush at mealtimes. To cut your calorie influx, then, slow down your eating and take time to chew your food. That way, you'll let your brain chemicals work their magic.

A rise in blood-sugar levels also signals your brain to stop eating. This triggers a release of insulin, which in turn increases levels of the brain messenger serotonin. Serotonin makes you feel 'sated' after a meal and so switches off hunger signals.

Long-term signals

Your fat cells produce a chemical signal called leptin that acts as a sort of 'fat thermostat' to keep body-fat levels at a constant and healthy level. If you put on extra fat, more leptin is produced, signalling the brain to reduce your appetite and increase your calorie output (by increasing your metabolic rate). If your fat levels dip too low, low leptin levels drive up your appetite, reduce your metabolic rate and signal your brain to eat.

Unfortunately, in practice, this leptin system doesn't always work perfectly – it is better at stopping people losing weight than gaining it. Scientists believe that it evolved during an age of food scarcity (rather than one of plenty) to warn of low body weight and thus ensure the body is fit to carry out essential functions like growth and reproduction. In other words, if the body's energy (fat) stores dip too low, puberty is delayed or fertility is reduced. However, this leptin system is not very effective in helping people lose weight.

Studies with rats at Rockefeller University, New York, found that those with a defective 'obese' gene gorge themselves into a state of obesity. Scientists believe that people who have this gene defect may have a breakdown in their leptin signalling mechanism – their brains do not receive the correct signals from the body's fat stores. This is called leptin resistance. Most obese people have high levels of leptin; it's just that their brains don't receive and respond to leptin signals. It may help explain why some people, despite having ample energy (fat) reserves, have a huge appetite. But the good news is that as you lose weight your cells become more sensitive and responsive to leptin again.

> Some people produce too much insulin, which means serotonin is not released in the normal manner. They don't get that after-meal 'glow' of satiety and can still feel hungry after eating.

The hunger-on switches

When your stomach is empty it produces the hunger-stimulating hormone ghrelin. Ghrelin makes your body want to eat more. As you get hungry, levels rise, telling your hypothalamus that you need to eat. As you eat, ghrelin levels fall, telling your hypothalamus you are full and triggering feelings of satiety.

If you try to ignore hunger, ghrelin levels go up, sending even more signals to eat, overriding your willpower and sooner or later causing you to reach for the biscuit tin! The chemical vicious cycle only stops when you eat. When your stomach is full, very little ghrelin is produced, thus reducing your appetite. That's why so many diets don't work – it's impossible to fight the biology of your body.

Researchers at the University of Washington believe that ghrelin may have evolved to help us survive during times of famine. If you starve yourself, your body makes more ghrelin to replenish its fat stores.

In a perfect system, levels of ghrelin and leptin balance each other so you eat as much food as you need and stop eating when you've had enough. In theory, you should stay at the same weight through your adult life. But, in reality, the system doesn't work quite so well: most people put on half a pound to a pound a year over much of their adult lives, which translates to an excess intake of just ten calories a day – about the equivalent of half a teaspoon of sugar.

Whatever scientists discover, one thing is certain: the key to understanding *your* appetite is to be sensitive to your body's signals.

Why do I eat twice as much food as normal in the week before my period?

The reason many women feel extra hungry premenstrually is linked to falls in levels of oestrogen and serotonin. These hormones normally help keep a check on your appetite. According to researchers at the Institute of Food Research (IFR) in the UK, low levels of serotonin dampen your mood. When you feel low your perception and expectation of certain foods changes, so you reach for comfort foods to make you

feel better. Low serotonin levels loosen the restraint you would
normally exercise over foods you perceive to be fattening.
So, you tuck into a whole tub of ice cream; you give yourself
'permission' to finish a pack of chocolate biscuits; and you can
no longer say no to a family-sized bar of chocolate. All your
usual restraint goes out of the window. The IFR researchers
found that women who normally restrict their food intake feel
more hungry premenstrually than those women who do not
restrict their calories. However, once hormone levels rise at the
onset of your period, your appetite goes back to normal.

How to satisfy your appetite

The key to managing your appetite – and thus losing unwanted
pounds – is to keep leptin levels high and ghrelin levels low. In other
words, high satiety and low hunger. Just as you can control your
blood pressure or blood cholesterol by changing the foods you eat,
you can also control the satiety centre in your brain.

The key is to focus on foods that satisfy your appetite for the
longest time yet provide relatively few calories. The more satiated
you feel after a meal, the less food you will eat at the next one and
the longer you will keep hunger at bay. Your aim should be to eat
foods that produce maximum satiety for as few calories as possible.

Scientists have discovered that certain foods will produce greater
satiety than others for the same calorie intake. If you feel full for
longer, you'll eat fewer calories and lose weight. But if you don't feel
sated you get hungry and tend to snack or overeat more readily.

The science of satiety

The whole notion of satiety is a complex one. Australian researcher Dr Susanne Holt and her team at the University of Sydney devised a way to assess foods according to their ability to keep hunger pangs at bay for the longest time. They developed a tool – the **satiety index (SI)** – that ranks different foods on their ability to satisfy hunger.

The results of Holt's experiments were first published in the *European Journal of Clinical Nutrition* in 1995. In this study, volunteers were fed fixed-calorie portions of different foods under a perspex hood to minimise the influence of appearance. The volunteers then told the scientists what their appetite ratings were. After two hours they were allowed to eat from a buffet while the scientists measured how much they ate from a variety of other foods and checked their hunger rating.

Each food was rated according to how much other food was eaten later. Using white bread as the baseline of 100 they ranked 38 different foods. Foods scoring 100 are judged to be as satisfying as white bread, foods scoring higher than 100 are more satisfying and those under 100 less satisfying.

The results of this study are shown in the table on page 44.

In general, the more satisfying a food felt, the more effective it proved as a nibbling deterrent. The experiments demonstrated that foods with a high fat content created almost instant cravings for more of the same. Croissants, for example, had the lowest score of all the foods tested, even though people think of them as filling. The best thing to eat for satiety is potatoes, which scored a tremendous 323 – making it easily the most satisfying food tested.

And there were more surprising results. Foods regarded as healthy such as bananas and muesli turned out to be no more satisfying than white bread. Fatty foods, such as chocolate bars and biscuits, were not as satisfying as expected. Jellybeans scored higher than expected at 118 – beating muesli and yoghurt and almost the same as white pasta.

What is satiety?

At its simplest, satiety is a measure of how long the consumption of a particular food will stop you feeling hungry again. Foods high on the Satiety Index list such as potatoes and porridge keep hunger pangs at bay for longer, while those low on the scale, such as cakes and croissants, are more likely to have you reaching for the cookie jar sooner.

The Satiety Index

All are compared to white bread (100)

Croissant	47
Cake	65
Doughnuts	68
Mars bar	70
Peanuts	84
Yoghurt	88
Ice cream	96

Less satisfying

Muesli	100	More satisfying
White bread	100	
French fries	116	
Special K	116	
Bananas	118	
Cornflakes	118	
Jellybeans	118	
White pasta	119	
Cookies	120	
Crackers	127	
Brown rice	132	
Lentils	133	
White rice	138	
Cheese	146	
Eggs	150	
All-Bran	151	
Grain bread	154	
Popcorn	154	
Wholemeal bread	157	
Grapes	162	
Baked beans	168	
Beef	176	
Wholemeal pasta	188	
Apples	197	
Oranges	202	
Porridge	209	
White fish	225	
Potatoes	323	

Choose foods that are more likely to leave you satisfied

The idea is that if you eat mostly foods with a 'high satiety' rating — foods that are nutritious and also satisfy your hunger — you will feel full on fewer calories. Feeling full and satisfied while eating foods you like makes it much easier to lose those unwanted pounds. Select mostly foods with a satiety index greater than a hundred.

More whole grains means a smaller waistline

Eating plenty of whole grains can help you lose weight and also prevent you gaining it, according to a 2007 Australian study. The researchers examined the results of 556 scientific studies published in the last 25 years and concluded that people who ate a diet high in whole grains (such as wholemeal bread, cereals, rice and pasta), beans and lentils were more likely to have a lower body weight and a smaller waist circumference than those who ate fewer whole-grain foods. The reason? Their high fibre content makes them filling and satisfying so you go on to eat fewer calories overall.

Go for volume

The biggest influence on satiety is a food's sheer bulk. Scientists have found that people tend to eat the same amount of food regardless of food type. In other words, a large volume of food will stimulate the stretch receptors in your stomach and quell your appetite better than a smaller amount of a different food, regardless of the number of calories they contain. Fibre and water add bulk without adding calories, fill you up and turn the appetite signals off.

Fibre-rich fruit, vegetables, beans, fish and whole grains do a better job of satisfying your hunger than foods rich in fat, sugar and refined starch. Low-satiety foods, such as cakes, doughnuts and chocolate, are easy to overeat, empty from your stomach quickly, and leave you hungry again in a relatively short time.

So fill up with plenty of fruit and vegetables – they contain fibre and around 90 per cent water. Try starting your meal with a low-calorie soup, such as a vegetable soup. A 2007 study at Pennsylvania State University has shown that eating vegetable soup at the start of a meal makes people eat less overall, so rather than piling on the pounds, the addition of the extra course can actually help people to lose weight.

Fill up with fibre

Fibre-rich foods tend to be bulky. They include beans, lentils, whole-grain foods (such as wholemeal bread, wholemeal pasta, bran flakes, Weetabix, brown rice and porridge), fruits, vegetables and nuts. These foods are digested relatively slowly and stay in your stomach longer, which means you feel full for quite a while. Fibre expands in the gut; it acts like a sponge, absorbing and holding onto water as it passes through you. This helps explain why fruits and vegetables fill you up more quickly than, say, cheese and crisps.

Choose porridge (SI 209) instead of cornflakes (SI 188) and wholemeal bread (SI 157) instead of white bread (SI 100).

A study of almost 3,000 adults in the US showed that over a ten-year period the people eating the most fibre gained less weight than those with the lowest intake of fibre. Scientists conclude that high-fibre diets help promote weight loss.

Fibre also increases a food's 'chewing time' so that your body has time to register that you are no longer hungry. This will make you less likely to overeat and help you feel full for longer. Studies have shown that people who increased their fibre intake for four months ate fewer calories and lost an average of five pounds – with no dieting!

A meal based on kidney beans, wholemeal pasta, lentils or porridge will fill you up with relatively few calories and keep you feeling full for a long time.

Whole fruits are more filling than dried or puréed versions and vastly more filling than juice. You can eat an awful lot of apples, for example, without taking in a lot of calories. They make your stomach feel full just because they take up so much space. But a glass of apple juice probably wouldn't, even though it has the same number of calories. A glass of juice provides 120 calories but you would have to eat two and half apples for the same calories.

How to eat more fibre

- Include beans and lentils in your meals at least once a week, then gradually increase it to four times weekly or more. Use them for making dahl, soups, salads, curries and pilaffs. Add to Bolognese sauce, stews, chilli and shepherd's pie.

- Aim for at least five portions of fruit and vegetables a day. Carry fresh fruit with you to have as a snack when you feel peckish.
- Start the day with a bowl of porridge or breakfast cereals labelled whole grain, for example bran flakes, Shreddies, Shredded Wheat or Weetabix.
- Swap white bread for whole-grain breads, such as wholemeal, rye or oatmeal.
- Use whole grains in one-pot dishes, such as barley in vegetables or stews and bulgur wheat in casseroles or stir-fries. Create a whole-grain pilaff with a mixture of barley, wild rice, brown rice, stock and herbs. Then add toasted nuts or chopped dried fruit.

Cut fat

In theory, high-fat foods, because they are two and a half times as calorie-dense as protein or carbohydrate, should make you feel very full, and they do – but not instantly. Because of the ease with which we can eat large quantities of these foods, we often rely on the stretch receptors in our stomach to tell us when we have eaten too much high-fat food, rather than the psychological sense of fullness. It's easy to eat a lot of doughnuts, which are much less filling than bread and only one third as filling as an orange! By the time your stomach feels full it's too late – you've already overeaten!

Satisfying protein

Foods rich in protein are more satiating than carbohydrate- or fat-rich foods. Protein slows down digestion and increases your feeling of fullness. It helps to turn off the appetite signals. This is one explanation as to why some people find it easy to stick to high-protein low-carbohydrate diets.

A lot of health-conscious dieters, in their quest to lose weight, opt for low-fat meals such as salad sandwiches, a vegetable stir-fry or toast and jam. The problem is, these kinds of meals do not keep hunger at bay because they don't contain enough protein. They can leave you hungry again after a couple of hours and reaching for a snack. Add a protein source (e.g. vegetable and bean soup; chicken and salad sandwiches; or vegetable and tofu stir-fry) and you'll find that the meal will keep you satisfied for hours.

Scientists believe this appetite-dampening effect may be due to the action of one of the amino acids (building blocks) in protein – leucine – acting on the hypothalamus in the brain. Studies at the University of Cincinnati, US, found that rats given leucine ate one third fewer calories than those who were not given this amino acid.

In practical terms this means including a portion of a protein-rich food – such as fish, poultry, lean meat, beans, lentils, milk, cheese, yoghurt, soya or nuts – in each meal. This can make the meal more satisfying – baked beans on whole-grain toast is three times as filling as a croissant – and will help delay hunger. But don't overdo it – eating more protein than you need won't help you lose weight faster!

Also, this doesn't mean eating a high-protein or Atkins-style diet

– which can risk leading to kidney stones and bone thinning – rather including sensible portions of protein-rich foods in your meals.

GI or SI?

Researchers now believe that satiety ratings are a better reference point for evaluating foods for weight control than glycaemic index (GI). According to Barbara Rolls, Professor of Nutrition at Penn State University in the US, GI has very little effect on satiety, despite the claims made in GI diet books. The idea that foods with a low GI make you feel full longer and help you lose weight is not strictly true. Many foods with a low GI rating (e.g. cakes, muesli) have a low satiety rating, which means that they don't leave you feeling full. They also have a high calorie content for a relatively small volume (i.e. a high calorie density – see Chapter 3). Consequently, on low-GI diets (where you're encouraged to fill up on low-GI foods) you can easily end up consuming *more* calories, even though you think you're eating less!

How to curb your appetite and eat less

Thirsty or hungry?

Many people confuse thirst with hunger. Both thirst and hunger sensations are generated in the same part of the brain, the satiety centre, to indicate the brain's satiety needs. If you don't recognise the sensation of thirst, you may assume that you are hungry, so you eat instead of drinking water. Next time you're feeling peckish, drink a glass of water and wait ten minutes to see if you are still hungry.

Are you really hungry?

If you have no idea when you are hungry, don't eat, as it means you aren't hungry. On the other hand, don't wait until you are very hungry or starving before eating. Otherwise, ghrelin levels will soar and you will end up eating the wrong foods or overeating.

Get into a routine

Make an effort to schedule regular meals that fit around your hunger, not your daily commitments. Leading a busy, stressful life often causes your eating patterns to become haphazard. The result is you end up eating not when you're hungry but just because you have the opportunity. You can lose the ability to make the connection between true hunger and eating, and end up overeating.

Speed control

Eating your food slowly and in a relaxed state of mind will curb your desire to eat more than you need. According to research at the University of Florida, scoffing your meal means that the satiety centre in the brain doesn't receive the right signals and explains why you may feel hungrier sooner. Researchers at the University of

Rhode Island gave volunteers a pasta meal on two occasions, which they were asked to eat either quickly or slowly. When eating as fast as they could, the volunteers ate 67 more calories than on the slow occasion.

Cut your food into smaller pieces, chew each mouthful thoroughly and don't load your fork with more food before swallowing the previous mouthful. Try putting down your knife and fork between mouthfuls. Not only will it allow the natural process of satiety more time to work, but you'll also be able to savour the taste of your food more.

Sleep more

Sleeping an extra hour or so may help you lose weight. This may sound too good to be true but, according to a study published in the journal *Sleep* in 2004, those who slept nine hours or more had, on average, a significantly lower body mass index than those who slept five hours or less. A lack of sleep boosts levels of ghrelin (the hunger hormone), while lowering levels of leptin (which makes us feel full). This hormonal imbalance sends a signal to the brain that more food is needed when, in fact, enough has been eaten. Research at the University of Chicago also shows that sleeping for four hours or less increases levels of another hormone, cortisol, which makes you feel hungry in the evening rather than sleepy.

Enjoy eating

Eating should be a pleasurable experience, so make time to savour your food. When you sit down to eat, taste every mouthful and enjoy every bite. Stop eating the moment you stop savouring the food or the moment you are full. It's easier to notice you are full if you pay attention while you are eating. That way, your body sends you a message that it is satisfied. But if you don't concentrate while you eat, your body may be telling you it's full but you may override the feeling of fullness and overeat.

Fill your tank

Don't even think about skipping breakfast. People who do are more likely to overeat later in the day and pile on unwanted pounds. When you start your day off with a healthy, filling breakfast, you dramatically increase your chances of eating healthily throughout the day. You also fuel your body, so you feel happy and energised for the rest of the day. Studies show that when you eat a filling, high-fibre breakfast you'll eat 100 to 150 fewer calories for breakfast and lunch. Have a bowl of porridge or whole-grain toast with fruit; both are high in fibre.

Don't eat too many diet foods

Your body is clever at discovering what's in the food you eat and you can't fool it for long. If you eat food that looks like it should be high calorie or high fat but actually isn't (such as low-calorie cakes and biscuits), your body will soon cotton on.

Experiments show that once it realises a food's appearance and taste promises don't match up to its calorie properties your body adjusts your hunger response so you no longer feel satisfied eating that food. The calorie savings of many low-fat products are often small anyway, as sugar replaces most of the fat reduction.

Eat to the (slow) beat

Listening to relaxing music while you eat can help you lose weight. Studies at Johns Hopkins University in Baltimore, Maryland have found that listening to classical (or other relaxing) music while eating makes you chew more slowly and eat less than when listening to frantic tunes.

Don't nosh while you watch

Do you eat your dinner in front of the TV? A study by the US Department of Agriculture found that people who watched more than two hours of TV a day were heavier than those who watched less than one hour, consuming an extra 154 calories. The distraction of television postpones the point at which you stop eating. So always eat your meal at the table rather than having supper on the sofa. This way you can concentrate on the flavours and textures of the food and tune in to the signals that your body gives you. After a few meals like this you'll soon have a good idea of when you've eaten enough and so will be less prone to overeating.

Eat without distractions

When you're not concentrating on your meal it's harder to listen to your body and recognise when you are full. A study by French researchers concluded that you may be prone to putting on the pounds if you eat while doing something else. Researchers measured how much women ate for lunch under different conditions, including in silence, or listening to a story. It turned out that the women ate more food – an average 300 calories more – while listening to the story compared with eating in silence.

Don't skip your favourite foods

The moment you tell yourself you can't have something – whether it's chocolate, crisps, cake or whatever – you want it. Even if you eat other things, you'll still want that forbidden treat and eventually you'll give in and have it anyway. Including your favourite foods in moderation will make your weight-loss plan easier to stick to, if not pleasurable. If you know that you can eat a little of your favourite indulgence every day, you'll stop thinking of it as a forbidden food and then won't want to binge on it. So go ahead and include chocolate or ice cream, but make sure it's only a little. Studies have shown that your taste buds are satisfied after the first three or four bites.

Midway meal check

If you always clear your plate as a matter of course, you're not allowing your brain to work out how hungry you are. The chances are you'll inevitably overeat. If you're full, don't feel you have to finish every last morsel. It's OK to leave food on your plate.

Simplify your food choices

Research at Tufts University in Massachusetts shows that when people are presented with a wider variety of foods they eat considerably more. Also, when you eat a single food, your eating slows down, you are satiated more quickly and so you eat less. The pleasure of eating a food increases up to the third or fourth bite, and then drops off. If you have lots of different foods on your plate you prolong the sensory pleasure, which stops you feeling full. The message here is to simplify your diet. Place fewer types of food on your plate. When shopping, stick to your list and ignore the lure of new varieties of ready-made meals and snacks on the shelves.

Ignore peer pressure

When eating with others it's tempting to eat more than when you are alone. You're less likely to listen to your hunger cues and more tempted to have second helpings. One study found that people who dined in a group of two or more ate nearly twice as much on average as those who ate alone. Learn to say 'no' politely and stick to eating only what your hunger dictates you want, not what others encourage you to eat.

Curb evening nibbling

Do you find it easy to stick to low-calorie eating during the day, then end up overeating in the evening? Skipping breakfast or lunch (or eating only small amounts) may seem an easy way of saving calories, but not meeting your energy needs during the day and then back-loading at night is the perfect scenario for gaining fat. Levels of hunger hormones rise through the day, leading to an overwhelming desire for food in the evening. Aim to eat two thirds of your day's total calories before your evening meal. Eating more, earlier, will cage those late-night hunger demons.

Avoid high-fructose corn syrup

Eating products containing high-fructose corn syrup (HFCS) can make you fat and upset your appetite-suppressing hormones, making overeating more likely. Fructose isn't broken down into energy in the same way as ordinary sugar. Instead, it is transported to the liver, where it is converted into fat. Studies at the University of Minnesota in the US found that people who regularly consumed HFCS had dramatically higher levels of fat in their blood, and an elevated risk of diabetes and heart disease. It seems to switch the body from fat-burning to fat-storage mode, according to University of California research in 1995. Look for HFCS – also called glucose fructose syrup – on labels of items such as soft drinks, biscuits, ice cream, sauces and frozen desserts. It's a cheap alternative to sugar used to help extend the shelf life of food.

Slim secret no. 3
Eat More for Less

Diets fail for various reasons but one of the reasons people give up is that they feel hungry and deprived all the time. It may sound an obvious point, but it's one that's overlooked by most diet plans. If you're hungry, you're more likely to break the diet 'rules' and eat whatever takes your fancy in order to quell your hunger. So you regain your weight and the vicious cycle goes on. The key is to keep portion sizes the same (or bigger) and simply change the balance of the types of foods you eat. In this chapter you'll learn how to make food choices that help you feel full with fewer calories. So you'll literally eat more for less (calories). Weight-loss researchers now focus on the calorie density of foods. The third secret to successful weight loss is to eat more foods with a low calorie density.

What is calorie density?

Scientists have found that people eat about the same weight of food each day. Although you may eat a different number of calories from day to day, the amount (weight) of food you eat stays surprisingly similar. It seems as if we have learned, over time, to satisfy our appetite with a certain amount of food. To feel full and satisfied, the secret is to choose foods that contain the least amount of calories in the biggest portion. In other words, foods with a low calorie density.

The calorie density tells you how many calories are in each gram of a particular food.

How to calculate calorie density

To work out a food's calorie density, read the label and then divide the number of calories in a serving by its weight in grams.

The formula to use is:

$$\textbf{Calorie density} = \frac{\textbf{calories (per portion)}}{\textbf{grams (per portion)}}$$

For example, suppose you have a 125g pot of yoghurt providing 130 calories per pot:

$$\textbf{Calorie density} = \textbf{130} \div \textbf{125} = \textbf{1.04}$$

Foods with a high calorie density provide a lot of calories per gram, while foods with a low calorie density contain relatively few calories for the same weight of food.

So, the secret to cutting your calories without cutting the *amount* of food you eat is to cut the calorie density of your diet. Aim to select mostly foods with a calorie density less than 1.5 (see accompanying table on calorie density of foods). Eat foods with higher calorie densities less often or in smaller portions. This will allow you to feel full on fewer calories – and lose weight!

As a rule of thumb:

- If the calories are fewer than the grams, the calorie density is less than 1. So go ahead, enjoy satisfying portions!
- If the calories are almost the same as the grams, the calorie density is about 1. OK, but exercise portion control!
- If the calories are double the grams, the calorie density is about 2, and if the calories are more than twice the grams, the calorie density is greater than 2. Keep a close eye on portion size!

Your aim, then, is to choose foods or meals that have fewer calories in your usual portion size. This way you will be able to satisfy your appetite with fewer calories, you won't have to cut down the amount you eat and – best of all – you won't feel hungry.

For example, swapping a square of chocolate (20g) for a large banana (100g) gives you a much bigger portion size for the same number of calories (95 calories). The banana has a much lower calorie density than the chocolate (1.0 against 5.2) and is more filling. In general, high-fat foods, such as chocolate and cheesecake, also have a low satiety rating as well as a high calorie density.

Foods with a low calorie density (0–1.5 calories per gram) in ascending order, lowest first:

Coffee/tea	0.02	Broccoli	0.24
Cucumber	0.10	Spinach	0.25
Salad greens/lettuce	0.12	Cauliflower	0.28
Melon	0.13	Milk (skimmed)	0.32
Cabbage	0.14	Peppers	0.32
Tomatoes	0.17	Onions	0.36
Carrots	0.22	Pears	0.40
Green beans	0.22	Milk (semi-skimmed)	0.46
Apples	0.47	Pasta	0.86
Yoghurt (virtually fat-free)	0.47	Bananas	0.95
Vegetable soup	0.48	White fish (grilled, baked or poached)	0.96
Tomato soup	0.52	Sorbet	0.97
Grapes	0.56	Prawns	0.99
Yoghurt (plain)	0.56	Tuna (canned in brine)	0.99
Milk (whole)	0.66	Lentil soup	0.99
Peas	0.69	Cottage cheese	1.0
Rice pudding (low fat)	0.71	Lentils	1.0
Potatoes (boiled)	0.72	Vegetable lasagne	1.0
Yoghurt (low-fat fruit)	0.78	Potatoes (baked)	1.1
Baked beans	0.81	Sweet corn	1.1
Porridge (made with milk and water)	0.83	Chickpeas	1.2
		Rice	1.2

Foods with a medium calorie density (1.5–4.0 calories per gram) in ascending order, lowest first:

Eggs (boiled or poached)	1.5	Bread (white)	2.4
Turkey (grilled)	1.5	Mozzarella	2.6
Potatoes (roast)	1.5	Pizza Jam	2.6
Salmon (tinned)	1.5	Bagels	2.7
Ice cream	1.5	Raisins	2.7
Chicken tikka masala	1.6	Honey	2.9
Oven chips	1.6	Bacon (grilled)	2.9
Dried apricots	1.6	French fries	3.1
Chicken (grilled)	1.7	Brie	3.2
Eggs (fried)	1.8	Bran flakes	3.3
Steak (grilled)	1.9	Bacon (fried)	3.5
Lasagne	1.9	Muesli	3.7
Avocado	1.9	Jaffa Cakes	3.8
Chapatis (without fat)	2.0	Sweets	3.8
Bread (wholemeal)	2.2	Cornflakes	3.8
Hamburger	2.4	Low-fat spread	3.9
Chips	2.4		

Foods with a high calorie density (more than 4.0 calories per gram) in ascending order, lowest first:

Sugar	4.0	Tortilla chips	4.6
Crackers	4.1	Biscuits	4.6
Oatcakes	4.1	French dressing	4.6
Cheese (cheddar)	4.1	Cereal bar	4.7
Cheesecake	4.3	Chocolate cake	4.8
Crisps (low fat)	4.6	Sponge cake	4.9

Chocolate biscuits	4.9	Peanuts	6.0
Flapjacks	4.9	Almonds	6.1
Shortbread	5.1	Mayonnaise	6.9
Chocolate	5.2	Butter	7.4
Crisps	5.3	Margarine	7.4
Reduced-fat spread	5.7	Olive oil	9.0
Peanut butter	6.0		

The calorie density of foods – a summary

Low calorie density 0.6–1.5 Eat larger portions	Most fruits (e.g. strawberries, apples, oranges), non-starchy vegetables (e.g. carrots, broccoli), salad vegetables (e.g. lettuce, cucumber), skimmed milk, clear soups, fat-free or plain yoghurt, starchy vegetables (e.g. sweet corn, potatoes), low-fat fruit yoghurt, pulses (beans, lentils and peas), pasta, rice and other cooked grains, breakfast cereals with low-fat milk
Medium calorie density 1.5–4.0 Eat moderate portions	Meat, poultry, lower-fat cheeses, eggs, pizza, chips (fries), raisins, salad dressings, bread, ice cream, cake
High calorie density 4.0 and over Eat small portions or substitute low-fat versions	Crackers, crisps, chocolate, sweets, croissants, biscuits, cereal bars, nuts, butter and oils

How to lower the calorie density of your diet

To lower the calorie density of a meal, eat larger portions of foods with a low calorie density (less than 1.5) but keep a tighter rein on portions of calorie-dense foods.

Foods like fruit, vegetables, beans, lentils and low-fat dairy products will provide you with satisfying portions for relatively few calories. However, foods such as bread, pasta, cereals, meat, poultry and dried fruit should be eaten in slightly smaller portions, and foods such as cheese, crisps, chocolate, biscuits, cereal bars, nuts and butter should be eaten in smaller portions still. The idea is that you lower the calorie density of your diet by cutting back on calorie-dense foods, while increasing the volume of your diet with foods with a low calorie density. In this way you still get to eat your normal weight or volume of food and feel satisfied.

Veg out

You can lower the calorie density of a dish or meal by adding water-rich ingredients such as vegetables, salad or fruits (water has a calorie density of zero) and cutting down portion sizes of higher-fat foods. By increasing the amount of vegetables and fruit in a meal you can have satisfying portions for relatively few calories.

At mealtimes, try replacing half of your usual portion of meat or pasta dish with vegetables such as carrots, broccoli, green beans or cauliflower. That way you won't feel like you're eating less.

Add extra vegetables to sauces, soups and stews as 'stealth' vegetables. Not only will they lower the calorie content of the portion you eat, but they will also boost the nutritional content of the meal.

- Think of your plate as a clock and allot at least 30 'minutes' of it to salad, vegetables and fruits.
- Stuff salad vegetables in everything you eat: sandwiches, rolls and wraps. Stir green veg (e.g. broccoli florets, spinach and cabbage) into soups, curries and hotpots.
- Add extra vegetables to as many dishes as possible: sauces, soups, curries and hotpots. Add chopped carrots, mushrooms and peppers to pasta sauce; add root vegetables, butternut squash and cauliflower to soup; bulk out the sauce in lasagne with grated carrots and courgettes; add extra peppers or broccoli to hot stews, bakes and pies.
- If you don't always have time to chop vegetables, use pre-prepared or frozen varieties instead. Many frozen vegetables such as peas are just as nutritious as fresh versions as they're frozen within hours of picking.
- Have a salad or dish of fruit as a starter. This can cut the number of calories you eat in your main meal by 12 per cent, according to a 2004 study published in the *Journal of the American Dietetic Association*. All that fibre and water takes the edge off your appetite so you eat less of the higher-calorie foods.
- For breakfast, start with an orange, a grapefruit, some berries or a sliced banana, then move on to yoghurt, toast or cereal. The fruit will fill you up and help keep hunger pangs at bay until lunchtime.

- Eating more fruit is one of the best things you can do for your health. Aim for two to four daily portions. Apart from the vital vitamins and minerals they provide, scientists know that fruit (and veg) contain a whole armoury of other useful substances that can protect you from heart disease and stroke, helping you lead a healthier and longer life.
- Instead of pudding, try stewed apples or plums with a spoonful of yoghurt, fruit kebabs (threaded onto wooden skewers), fruit with low-fat custard, baked apples, baked bananas, fresh or tinned fruit mixed with yoghurt, rice pudding with fresh raspberries, and apple crumble.

Hiding veg helps cut calories

In a study of 61 children at Pennsylvania State University, researchers provided two pasta sauces, one of which included broccoli and cauliflower blended into the sauce, which reduced the calorie content per portion by a quarter. The researchers found children who ate the pasta with the lower-calorie sauce consumed 17 per cent fewer calories overall. What's more, the children could not tell the difference and ate a consistent amount of pasta.

Eat less fat

Fat provides a lot of calories for a very small weight. It provides nine calories per gram, twice as many as carbohydrate or protein (four

Slim Secrets

calories per gram). Its high calorie density (as well as its texture and ability to carry a food's flavours) means that it's easy to overeat.

So reducing the amount of fat you eat will lower the calorie density of your diet. It means you can eat bigger portions for the same or even fewer calories. One of the easiest ways to achieve this is by substituting reduced-fat or low-fat versions for high-fat dairy products (e.g. skimmed instead of whole milk; low-fat yoghurt for creamy yoghurt). You could switch to lower-fat cooking methods (e.g. grilling instead of frying), and experiment with non-fat flavouring ingredients for your food, e.g. onions, garlic, lemon zest, herbs and spices.

But don't cut fat out of your diet completely. You need a certain amount of 'good' fats (the unsaturated fats found in fish, nuts, seeds and their oils). Aim to minimise saturated fats (found in meat, butter and full-fat dairy products) and trans fats (found in hydrogenated and partially hydrogenated fats in, e.g., biscuits, cakes, desserts, crackers) – both can raise your blood cholesterol levels and increase your risk of heart disease.

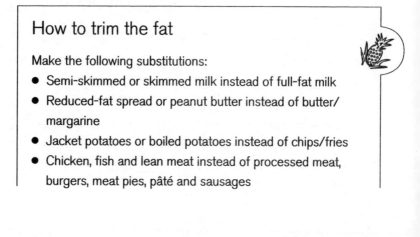

How to trim the fat

Make the following substitutions:
- Semi-skimmed or skimmed milk instead of full-fat milk
- Reduced-fat spread or peanut butter instead of butter/margarine
- Jacket potatoes or boiled potatoes instead of chips/fries
- Chicken, fish and lean meat instead of processed meat, burgers, meat pies, pâté and sausages

- Crackers, rice cakes and fruit bars instead of biscuits and cakes
- Fresh fruit instead of desserts, chocolate and cakes
- Heart-healthy monounsaturated oils (e.g. olive oil), spreads and nuts instead of butter, cooking fats and margarine containing hydrogenated fats

Use lower fat cooking methods:
- Skip pre-frying onions when making soups, hotpots and stews; add them to the pan with the other ingredients, including the liquid, and cook as normal
- Make sauces without butter by blending cornflour and milk, then add to the rest of the milk and bring to the boil
- Limit frying except stir-frying, using only minimal amounts of oil
- Boiling, steaming, grilling and stir-frying are healthier ways to cook your food
- You don't have to give up frying altogether – using a one-cal spray instead of a teaspoon of oil saves about 50 calories
- Add yoghurt instead of cream to sauces (but don't let it boil)

Flavour your food without fat:
- Top baked potatoes with fromage frais, yoghurt, a little pesto or baked beans
- Rather than use mayonnaise and oily dressings, have salads with low-fat salad dressings, balsamic or flavoured vinegars, or low-fat yoghurt seasoned with fresh herbs, lemon or lime juice

- Add flavour with fat-free condiments such as mustard, herbs, herb salt, soy sauce and salsa

Is it true that drinking a glass of water before a meal fills you up and makes you eat less?

The answer is no. Drinking water fills you only temporarily, but as it contains no fibre or nutrients it passes straight through your stomach quickly. It won't satisfy your appetite or make you eat less at mealtimes.

Drinking a glass of water with your meal won't necessarily fill you up more or satisfy your appetite either. That's because the stomach sieves the water from the food, allowing it to pass quickly from your stomach into the intestines.

However, if you combine the water and food in a soup this sieving is prevented. The water and the nutrients from the food stay mixed together in your stomach for longer, activating your satiety signals and delaying emptying, which can reduce your hunger by up to a quarter.

Eat less sugar

Sugar adds extra calories without extra bulk. In other words, it increases the calorie density of a food. In general, sugary foods don't fill you up or satisfy your hunger.

When you eat a sugar-rich food you get a rapid boost to blood-sugar levels. You experience a surge of energy as the sugar reaches the bloodstream and your brain receptors are told that food energy has arrived. But insulin is quickly released into the bloodstream to dampen down that excess sugar, converting it to glycogen or fat. This sudden drop in blood-sugar levels makes you feel hungry again. So, after the initial 'rush', sugary foods deliver the double whammy of adding to your fat stores while leaving you hungry.

What's more, foods such as cakes, biscuits, desserts, chocolate, sweets and sugar-rich drinks generally provide very low levels of essential nutrients.

Avoiding sugary foods or reducing the amount of sugar you add to food and drinks will reduce the calorie density of your diet.

Here are some ways to help you cut down:

- Swap sugary desserts for fresh fruit, a bowl of yoghurt topped with strawberries, blueberries or sliced banana, or try one of the recipes in this book (see page 201). For many people a sweet dessert signals to your brain that the meal is over. Without it, you may not feel satisfied, which might leave you raiding the fridge later on for something to satisfy your sugar craving.
- Substitute honey for sugar in cooking. It saves calories as well as adding antioxidants to protect your heart and health. It's sweeter than sugar (on average up to 50 per cent sweeter) so, for cooking or adding to drinks, you need to use less. The American Chemical Society reports that honey contains substances that can help protect against cancer and ageing.
- When you fancy something sweet, opt for foods that are also

rich in fibre and/or water such as delicious fruits – think berries, oranges, grapes, apricots, apples, plums, nectarines and cherries.

- Swap sugar-rich drinks for calorie-free alternatives. The average person consumes 14 per cent of their daily calories in liquid form – sugary fizz, alcoholic drinks and hot drinks – so switching to water or herbal tea can save you more than 8,000 calories – equivalent to a weight loss of over 1kg (2lb) – every month.
- If you take sugar in hot drinks, or add sugar to your breakfast cereal, gradually reduce the amount until you can cut it out altogether.
- Check food labels and pick the foods with less added sugar or go for the low-sugar version. For guidance, 10g sugars or more per 100g is a lot of sugar (and gets a red light on the front of pack labels) 2g sugars or less per 100g is a little sugar (and gets a green light on the front of pack labels).
- Choose whole-grain breakfast cereals with zero sugar or low levels (less than 2g/100g) rather than those coated with sugar.

Can dieting slow down your metabolic rate?

Strict dieting will sabotage your efforts at weight control because it sends your body into 'famine' mode. Your body believes there is a food shortage so it adapts to the impending crisis by storing more calories as fat and burning fewer calories on essential processes, i.e. reducing the metabolic rate. This can be between 10 and 30 per cent depending how great the calorie drop is. However, the effect is not permanent as your

metabolic rate increases when your calorie intake increases.
Avoid a dramatic calorie cut – no more than around 15 per cent
is recommended – in order to avoid a metabolic slow-down.

Easy calorie swaps

Here are some easy ways to lose calories by opting for less calorie
dense alternatives:

Swap	For this	And save
2 fried eggs	2 poached eggs	66 calories
Meat lasagne (420g)	Vegetable lasagne (420g)	173 calories
1 chocolate biscuit	1 rice cake	100 calories
1 slice cheesecake	1 pot low-fat fruit yoghurt	122 calories
1 slice apple pie	Stewed apples with sugar (110g)	201 calories
1 bag crisps (30g)	30g plain popcorn	100 calories
1 flapjack	1 teacake	200 calories
2 crackers with 40g cheese	1 slice wholemeal toast with 1 tbsp low-fat cheese	107 calories
1 rasher streaky bacon	1 rasher trimmed back bacon	40 calories
1 croissant	30g bran flakes with semi-skimmed milk	67 calories
1 Mars bar	1 banana	180 calories
50g raisins	50g grapes	106 calories
Cappuccino	'Skinny' cappuccino	46 calories
Chicken korma (350g)	Chicken tikka (350g)	230 calories

Top satisfying secrets

Here are more ways to help avoid that empty feeling.

Choose foods that need chewing

Foods that take a little more effort to chew take longer to eat and hence are more filling. Chewing promotes satiety, partly because it slows down eating but also because it encourages the release of enzymes and hormones that register fullness in your brain.

Opt for whole fruit rather than smoothies and juices; add extra vegetables to dinner; bulk up soups/hotpots/curries with extra tinned beans and serve this with a bulky whole-grain bread.

Fill up with soup

Pennsylvania State University studies have found that starting your meal with a bowl of soup can cut your calorie consumption by 20 per cent compared with eating the main course alone. It doesn't matter whether you choose a chunky or a smooth/puréed soup, but it should be a low-calorie variety providing no more than 150 calories per portion (such as vegetable soup, which was tested in the studies) rather than a creamy one. The likely explanation is that the fibre and liquid fills your stomach, so you then go on to eat less food. Other studies at the University of Nottingham have shown that blending food to make a soup makes people feel full for longer than eating the same food and drinking a glass of water. It seems as if combining the food and liquid to make a soup takes up more volume and stays in the stomach for longer, so you feel full for longer.

Start with salad

Eating a large portion of foods with a low calorie density, such as salad, as a starter can cut the number of calories you eat in your main meal by 12 per cent, according to a 2004 study at Pennsylvania State University. All that fibre and water takes the edge off your appetite so you eat less of the higher-calorie foods. Take care not to add too much dressing, though.

Eat fruit first

Start breakfast with an orange, a grapefruit, some berries or a sliced banana, then move on to the rest. The fibre and water fill you up and satisfy your appetite for relatively few calories, and you'll get a healthy dose of vitamins. It's also an easy way to get one of your five-a-day portions. And it'll put you in a positive food mindset for the rest of the day.

Bar none

Don't be seduced by the healthy image or tempted by the health claims (such as 'only 90 calories', 'contains whole-grain goodness') of cereal and breakfast bars. Their calorie density is similar to those of biscuits or chocolate bars. The main difference is their smaller portion size. Most are deceptively high in sugar; typically around one third of their weight is in the form of glucose syrup, fructose, invert sugar, sucrose or brown sugar – all different types of sugars – which makes them quick to eat before they've filled you up. Their whole-grain cereal content is surprisingly low, which means the fibre content – and therefore satiety value – is also low. Most supply little more than 1g per bar – around 5 per cent of your daily fibre requirement – which is not much higher than a digestive biscuit. Some popular brands contain harmful hydrogenated oils, so check the ingredients list on the label carefully.

Don't bag it

Peckish? Avoid reaching for a bag of crisps (or any other bagged snack). These savoury snacks are very calorie dense – around 5.3 – which means they are very easy to overeat. By the time your brain registers you're full, you will have overeaten. They don't fill you up nor satisfy your appetite and – because of the high salt content – can actually make you hungrier and thirstier. Opt for fresh fruit, low-fat yoghurt or rice cakes instead.

Don't crush or squeeze

Both fruit juice and smoothies contain much higher concentrations of (natural) sugar than the fresh fruit they came from and are less satiating.

When you squeeze the fruit you lose the filling power of fibre. Even crushing it to make a smoothie destroys the cell walls, so you don't have to chew the fruit. This means it's easy to overconsume calories before your hunger is satisfied. Down a glass of orange juice and you'll take in about 120 calories, but if you eat an orange instead you'll save 60 calories, get more fibre and feel more satisfied.

Undress your salad

Salads can be low in calories but watch what you have with them. Croutons and salad dressings can quickly turn a low-calorie meal into a high-calorie one. Lose them from a Caesar salad and you'll save about 200 calories. Better still, have a leafy salad with lots of tomatoes, peppers, radishes, etc. with a small wholemeal roll and balsamic dressing.

Super-size your sarnie

Most pre-prepared sandwiches have a relatively high calorie density and poor filling power. Cut the calorie density and enjoy a more filling meal by opting for an open sandwich with extra salad (see recipes on page 206) or getting one made to order and ask for grilled vegetables or lots of tomato, avocado, rocket and watercress. It's a bigger lunch, too.

Beware of (some) low-fat foods

The title 'low fat' can be misleading. With milk and yoghurt, low fat is desirable, but with many other foods, the reduction in fat can be compensated by the addition of sugar or refined starch, neither of which you need to load up with. Only eat low-fat versions of foods if you like the taste: in many cases, low fat can equal low satisfaction for your taste buds. Low-fat foods may not always satisfy your taste expectations and you'll end up eating the high-fat version anyway. If you do opt for low-fat foods, keep portion sizes the same (it's tempting to allow yourself bigger portions!) and don't use them as an excuse to indulge in high-fat treats later on.

Do sugar-free drinks help you cut down on calories?

Researchers at the University of Australia gave volunteers equal amounts of sugar-rich cola, sugar-free cola and water in random order on separate mornings. The volunteers were then allowed free access to potato crisps 20 minutes later followed by a buffet lunch. The amount of calories they ate after each of the three drinks was no different. So the calorie-free drink did not help people cut down their daily calorie intake.

Putting it into practice . . .

Breakfast ideas

Porridge with sliced bananas (whole oats are more filling than instant porridge)
or
Bran-enriched cereal with skimmed milk and fresh fruit

or

Wholemeal toast (with a little honey) plus oranges/satsumas

Lunch ideas

Large bowl of vegetable or lentil soup with wholemeal roll; low-fat yoghurt

or

Open wholemeal sandwich with tuna and grilled vegetables plus extra salad; grapes

or

Baked potato with hummus or ratatouille and salad; apple

Supper ideas

Grilled chicken breast served with brown rice, broccoli and cauliflower

or

Fish with spicy chickpeas

or

Lentil and vegetable curry with brown rice

or

Red kidney bean and vegetable hotpot with boiled or baked potatoes

or

Wholemeal pasta primavera (tomato sauce with courgettes, peppers, peas)

or

Chilli made with red kidney beans, lean mince, carrots, peppers, tomatoes and courgettes with brown rice

Snack ideas

Fresh fruit, popcorn, low-fat yoghurt, wholemeal toast, vegetable crudités

Slim secret no. 4
Manage Your Portions

Knowing which foods will satisfy your appetite best or fill you up for the fewest calories will definitely help you manage your weight. But the biggest weight-loss challenge is knowing exactly how much you should be eating.

Have you noticed how easy it is to eat a giant bowl of pasta in a restaurant, a portion several times larger than one you would normally serve yourself at home? And how easy it is to get through a massive chocolate muffin in a high street coffee shop? Or a bucket of popcorn at the cinema big enough to feed a family of four? With all that comes the risk of eating too many calories.

Most people typically think they are eating fewer – and burning more – calories than they really are. In general, people will underestimate the calories in an average meal by about 20 per cent. Why are we so far off the mark? Well, there are several factors at work, including your inability to accurately estimate portions, external cues that cause you to overeat, and difficulties gauging your daily calorie budget. Any one of these factors – or a combination of them – can be enough to thwart your best weight-loss efforts.

This chapter reveals some simple ways to control your portions (without feeling deprived) and your calorie intake.

Portion distortion

Research published in the *Journal of the American Dietetic Association* in 2006 shows that people's ideas of normal portion sizes have grown in the last twenty years. Restaurants dish out bigger portions than ever before and food manufacturers sell larger packs of snack foods at discount prices. For example, portions of orange juice served in restaurants have increased by more than 40 per cent in the last 20 years. In nutritional terms, this larger amount of orange juice provides an extra 50 calories, which equates to a 5lb (2kg) gain over the course of a year if you drank one a day.

Even foods like pizzas, rolls, crisps, ready-meals and scones are constantly growing in size. For example, a typical packet of crisps in the 1980s used to weigh 25g. Now a standard packet weighs 40–50g, giving you an extra 80–100 calories.

In the US study, people served themselves nearly 20 per cent more cornflakes and poured almost 30 per cent more milk on their cereal than people 20 years ago. More than half of the people in the study selected portions at breakfast larger than the 'standard' size. And 70 per cent selected larger-than-standard portions at lunch and dinner.

When you are served bigger meals in restaurants and buy bigger pack sizes in supermarkets your perception of what is an 'acceptable' amount to consume increases. It's easy to up the size of the portions you serve yourself at home without realising. If you base your portions on what you are served in restaurants you will be getting more calories than you need.

The problem, according to studies at Penn State University in the US, is you are unlikely to compensate for those extra calories by eating less later on. You will almost certainly overconsume calories over the day. It only takes a few hundred extra calories eaten here and there over a typical day to tip the balance from weight loss to weight gain. For example, one extra chocolate biscuit and one glass of wine a day over a year adds up to an excess 73,000 calories – which equates to a weight gain of 18lb (8kg). Very often these extra calories come from eating larger portions of everyday foods without noticing.

Clearly, portions have become distorted, and it's no surprise that people's waistlines have expanded.

How portions have got bigger

Researchers at the University of North Carolina in the US studied the changes in portion sizes in the US between 1977 and 1996. They found that portion sizes for many calorie-dense foods grew dramatically over that time. The amount of salty snacks increased by 93 calories per portion, soft drinks by 49 calories, hamburgers by 97 calories and French fries by 68 calories.

The eating-out conundrum

It's tempting to opt for those larger restaurant meals based on the notion that more food for the same money equals better value. But you would be short-changing your health and your waistline. The bigger portions that restaurants serve make people vulnerable to overeating because most people eat all or most of what is served. Indeed, a study at Penn State University found that bigger restaurant portions result in a higher calorie intake. In this study the size of a pasta dish was varied between a standard portion and a portion 50 per cent larger. Customers who ordered the meal were asked to rate their satisfaction and the appropriateness of the portion size.

The results showed that customers who were served the larger portion ate nearly all of it – consuming an extra 172 calories. The survey responses showed that the customers rated the size of both portions equally appropriate for meeting their needs. So, if you don't want to eat more than you need, steer clear of supersizing.

Can you get used to bigger portions?

In a Penn State University study, researchers found that when portion sizes of all foods served over a two-day period were increased, people continued to eat more at each meal. In other words, they didn't compensate for overeating the first day by cutting back on meals the next day. When portion sizes were 50 per cent bigger, the women in the study ate 335 more calories per day and the men 513 more calories. When the portion sizes were doubled, the women ate 530 calories more per day, the men 803 more. It didn't matter how much they had eaten the day before. Given more food, they ate more. They didn't compensate for having overeaten the day before.

Double trouble: high-calorie bigger portions

The worst combination is calorie-dense foods served in bigger portions. According to a 2003 Penn State University study big portions of calorie-dense food boost calorie intake further without providing greater satisfaction.

In this study 39 normal weight and overweight women ate breakfast, lunch and dinner once a week for six weeks in the University's Laboratory for the Study of Human Ingestive Behavior. The breakfasts and dinners were served in standard portions but the lunch was varied in portion size and calorie density. Portion size alone increased calorie intake by 20 per cent. Calorie density alone increased intake by 26 per cent. Together portion size and calorie density increased calorie intake by 56 per cent.

But the good news is that people still feel satisfied when given less. When people were given smaller portions and/ or less-calorie-dense meals, amazingly it didn't leave them hungry. Even though the volunteers ate 221 fewer calories when given the smaller meal of lower calorie density, they felt just as full and satisfied as when they had eaten the larger meal of higher calorie density.

All this suggests that lowering the calorie density of your meals will allow you to eat satisfying portions without consuming too many calories, which, in turn, allows you to manage your weight.

What makes you overeat?

In chapter 2, you learned how your body tells you when you've had enough. But it's easy to ignore and override these signals. For example, when you are presented with more food on your plate than meets your needs, you will probably eat more without even thinking about it.

A 2005 experiment at Cornell University in the US revealed that the size of a container can powerfully and unknowingly increase how much food a person consumes. Volunteers were given either a medium (120g) or large (240g) box of popcorn while watching a film. The people who were given the large boxes ate a staggering 45 per cent more than those given the medium boxes – 100 more calories to be exact. Even if the popcorn was stale, the volunteers still ate 30 per cent more.

Drinking from a bigger cup also makes you drink more and consume more calories. A 2006 study at Penn State University found that when volunteers were given a larger serving of drink with a meal, they drank 50 per cent more and consumed up to 25 per cent more calories. They did not compensate for the extra calories in the drink by eating less. In other words, people do not adjust their food intake to account for the calories in their drink.

Why do people eat more? It could be that you assume the portion given to you is the 'right' size. Or it could be that you are conditioned to finish everything that's on your plate. Perhaps you don't like to see food wasted or you were taught as a child to finish your plate.

In another study at Cornell University, volunteers were given bowls of soup and told to have as much as they wanted. However, unknown to them, some volunteers were given self-filling bowls, which refilled slowly as the volunteers ate. Amazingly, the people who had the self-filling bowls ate 73 per cent more soup than the others. This suggests that people tend to eat more if they see more food in front of them.

Your surroundings can also make you eat more. If you are distracted, watching the television or playing a game for example, you are more likely to eat beyond your needs. A study in the *British Journal of Nutrition* found that eating while distracted leaves you feeling less satisfied. Women given five Jaffa Cakes while playing a computer game said they felt less full after eating the biscuits and wanted more, while women given the same amount of biscuits without any distraction felt sated.

Being presented with a variety of food, rather than a single type, can make you eat more. Research at Tufts University in Massachusetts shows that when people are presented with a wider variety of foods they eat considerably more. Also, when you eat a single food, your eating slows down, you are satiated more quickly and so you eat less. The pleasure of eating a food increases up to the third or fourth bite, and then drops off. If you have lots of different foods on your plate you prolong the sensory pleasure, which stops you feeling full. The message here is to simplify your diet. Place fewer types of foods on your plate.

Hide the snacks

You're more likely to munch snacks if they are within sight and easy reach. In a study at Cornell University, New York, researchers put thirty chocolates in either clear or opaque dishes for office workers. The dishes were placed in four different ways: on their desks and visible; on their desks but in containers with lids so the chocolates weren't visible; about two metres away and visible; the same distance away but not visible. People ate eight chocolates a day when the bowl was on their desks and visible; they ate four chocolates a day when it was on their desk but covered. They ate five chocolates when the bowl was placed two metres away and visible but only three chocolates a day when it was the same distance away and not visible. It's a case of 'out of sight, out of mind'. The less visible and the less convenient the snacks, the less you'll think about them and be tempted to eat them.

Do you underestimate your calorie intake?

Most women think they eat fewer calories than they actually do. Researchers at the University of South Carolina compared the amount of food 100,000 women said they were eating and the amounts they would need according to their weight, height and metabolic levels. They found that women under-reported their calorie intake by 400 calories. One in four women under-reported by more than 800 calories. The more overweight the women were, the more calories they under-reported.

What is a portion?

Here is a guide to help you estimate portion sizes (scale up or down if you have small/big hands).

One cupped hand = 1 portion (80g) of vegetables
Two cupped hands = 1 portion (80g) of salad
Size of a tennis ball = 1 portion (80g) of fruit, e.g. apple, peach
One cupped hand = 1 portion (80g) of berries or chopped fruit
Size of a tennis ball = 1 portion (150g) of potatoes
Two cupped hands = 1 portion (40g) breakfast cereal flakes
One small cupped hand = 1 portion (25g) nuts or seeds
Deck of cards = 1 portion (85g) cooked meat or fish
Size of 4 dice = 1 portion (25g) cheese
One generous cupped hand = 1 portion (40g dry weight) pasta
One cupped hand = 1 portion (30g dry weight) rice
200ml glass or cup = 1 portion of milk or fruit juice

How many calories do you need?

Once you've got a good idea of portion sizes you can work out how many calories you should be eating every day, a number that depends on your age, gender, height, weight and activity level (for a simple calculator visit www.healthstatus.com).

Alternatively, you can estimate your daily calorie needs by working out your basal metabolic rate (BMR) and multiplying it by your physical activity level.

Your BMR is the number of calories you burn at rest over 24 hours, maintaining essential functions such as respiration, digestion and brain function. It accounts for 60 to 75 per cent of the calories you burn daily.

Step 1: Estimate your basal metabolic rate (BMR)

(A) Quick method: As a rule of thumb, BMR uses 11 calories for every half-kilo (1lb) of a woman's body weight and 12 calories per half kilo (1lb) of a man's body weight.

Women: BMR = weight in kilos × 2 × 11
(or weight in pounds × 11)

Men: BMR = weight in kilos × 2 × 12
(or weight in pounds × 12)

E.g., the BMR for a 60kg woman = 60 × 2 × 11 = 1,320 calories

(B) Longer method: For a more accurate estimation of your BMR, use the following equations:

Age	Men	Women
10–18	(weight in kg × 17.5) + 651	(weight in kg × 12.2) + 746
18–30	(weight in kg × 15.3) + 679	(weight in kg × 14.7) + 479
31–60	(weight in kg × 11.6) + 879	(weight in kg × 8.7) + 829
60+	(weight in kg × 13.5) + 487	(weight in kg × 10.5) + 596

E.g., the BMR for a 60kg woman aged 31–60 = (60 × 8.7) + 829 = 1,351 calories

Step 2: Estimate your physical activity level (PAL)

Your physical activity level (PAL) is the ratio of your overall daily energy expenditure to your BMR – a rough measure of your lifestyle activity:

- Mostly inactive or sedentary (mainly sitting): PAL = 1.2
- Fairly active (include walking and exercise once or twice a week): PAL = 1.3
- Moderately active (exercise two or three times weekly): PAL = 1.4
- Active (exercise hard more than three times weekly): PAL = 1.5
- Very active (exercise hard daily): PAL = 1.7

Step 3: Multiply your BMR by your PAL to work out your daily calorie needs

So, for example the daily energy needs for an active 60kg woman:

BMR × PAL = 1,351 × 1.5 = 2,027 calories

That's how many calories you burn a day to maintain your weight.

To *lose weight*, reduce your daily calorie intake by 15 per cent or multiply the figure above (your maintenance calorie needs) by 0.85. This will produce a fat loss of about half a kilo (1lb) per week.

E.g., the daily energy needs for an active 60kg woman to lose weight = 2,027 × 0.85 = 1,723 calories

Once you have determined how many calories you should be eating daily, you can divide that throughout the day to decide how much to eat at each meal.

How to stop eating too much

Here are some practical strategies to help you manage portions.

Fill your plate right

Treat meat-based dishes as side dishes rather than the main part of your meal. Load up on vegetables, salad and fresh fruit instead of using them as side dishes. Aim to cover at least two thirds of your plate with these foods. You'll feel full sooner and get extra vitamins and fibre. The higher the calorie density, the smaller the portion.

Listen to your body

Before you sit down to eat, get in touch with your true hunger. Try to gauge how much food your body really needs. Respond to your body's needs and simply eat the amount that is right for you. This may take practice but you will soon become attuned to your body's needs and learn to eat appropriate portions of food.

Bigger is not better

Restaurant and fast-food portions are oversized. Don't add insult to injury by 'going large', even if it seems better value. Larger portions only lead to higher calorie intake. Steer clear of meal deals altogether. Order larger or extra portions of vegetables and salads; starter-size portions of main courses; and don't be embarrassed to leave food on your plate once you've eaten enough.

Educate yourself about portion sizes

Just how many biscuits (or your other favourite snacks) are in a serving? Check the packet – you may be surprised at how many portions you are actually eating.

Familiarise yourself with what a standard portion looks like on your plate. This will help you manage portions when eating out or when you have less control over how much is served. As a rough guide, a portion of meat, poultry or fish (85g) is the size of a deck of cards; a portion of pasta, rice or potatoes looks like a tennis ball (see What is a Portion? page 89). Spend some time in the kitchen weighing and measuring foods. Work out how much you normally eat and the calories in these portions.

Downsize that dinner!

Don't be afraid to ask if you can purchase the lunch-size dish at dinner time. Many restaurants offer lunch-size portions of their dishes, which are smaller than their full-size dinner dishes. Or ask to order from the children's menu! Kids' meals contain what *used* to be normal-sized portions for us grown-ups.

If you tell your server that you're dieting, they'll probably allow it. Practising this portion-control tip will save your waistline some inches and your wallet a few pounds too!

Beware flat foods

Be extra careful when you order 'flat' foods, such as pizza, quiche or pancakes. A study at Rutgers University, New Jersey, found that people were more likely to underestimate portion sizes for flat foods, and overestimate portion sizes for thick, high foods such as cake!

Keep the evidence

If you want to eat less, try and keep some reminder of how much you have been munching. Research carried out at Cornell University, New York State, showed that if you have evidence of how much you've eaten it will deter you from eating more. Don't throw the packaging or wrappers in the bin straight away; keep the evidence around until you have finished eating.

Put leftovers out of sight

To avoid overeating at mealtimes, serve your portion and then put any leftovers out of sight – don't have the dish on the table in front of you. Try eating it in a different room – there will be less temptation to keep refilling your plate. That gives you more time to think, 'Am I still hungry?' or 'Do I really want another portion of pasta?' The answer in most cases is 'No.' Get into the habit of freezing leftovers or putting them in the fridge immediately, away from temptation.

Say no to seconds

If you have planned your meal properly and allowed yourself appropriate amounts of food, then second helpings mean a second meal. Stick to single servings.

Divide the pack

If you find your willpower is overpowered by large packs of calorie-dense foods such as nuts, crisps, cheese or biscuits, don't buy them! Alternatively, you can divide the contents into smaller portion sizes then wrap or store in smaller pots. That way you won't be tempted to eat more than you really need or finish off the pack in one go.

Buy small

In supermarkets, resist the temptation of jumbo packs and two-for-one offers for calorie-dense foods such as biscuits, desserts, ready-meals, scones, cakes and bakery items. You may tell yourself you'll only eat half the pack of crisps but the odds are you won't. Buy regular sizes or individually wrapped portions.

When you can't eat just one . . .

You've got a bag of sweets. How many do you eat? Well, that depends on how big the bag is, a study at the University of Illinois shows. When people were given a bag containing 114 M&Ms for a TV snack, they took an average 63 sweets (a total of 209 calories). But when they were given a bag with three times as many M&Ms, people took an average 103 M&Ms (a total of 341 calories). The bigger the bag, the more people ate. The advice is: if you're buying sweets or other calorie-dense foods, buy the smallest pack size or measure out your portion in a separate container then hide the rest.

Store food in portions

If you often make more food than you need, learn to cook less or divide the remainder into portions and keep in the fridge or freezer for later meals. Store them straight away to reduce temptation.

Keep temptation out of the way

It may sound obvious, but if you want to avoid the temptation of diet-wrecking snacks, don't bring them into your house. Although you may think you can control your consumption, it's a lot easier if the only things in the kitchen are fruit and vegetables, rather than crisps and biscuits.

Have a healthy snack before dining out

Do you sit down in a restaurant and can't decide what to eat? You want everything so end up ordering more than you could manage. If you've been feeling deprived it's hard to control your urge to make up for it. The combination of a wide choice of tempting foods and hunger can result in overeating. Avoid this by not letting yourself get too hungry. Have a small healthy snack, such as fruit or a rice cake with peanut butter before you go out so you won't be starving when it's time to order.

Don't be deceived by bite-sized snacks

Small may seem less risky but research has shown that it's easy to overindulge. People who were offered 6 regular-sized biscuits ate an average of 3, while those offered 25 mini-biscuits ate between 15 and 18 – consuming double the number of calories.

Measure up carefully

While the oft-quoted small glass of red wine at 85 calories doesn't sound too ruinous, in reality most bars and restaurants serve more generous-sized measures of 175ml (119 calories) and 250ml (170 calories). So, a couple of big glasses could cost you more than the calorie equivalent of a cheeseburger (299 calories). Similarly, trading up a half of draught lager (90 calories) for a 440ml can of the premium stuff (260 calories) and you'll be downing the calorie equivalent of a Mars bar.

Use a smaller plate

The size of the plate you eat from, the bowls you serve yourself from and the utensils you use can make you eat more than you think you do. Switching to eating from a smaller plate – making the amount you put on it look larger – means you will automatically eat at least 25 per cent less. Experiments in the US have found that when people serve themselves from bigger bowls and use larger serving spoons, they serve themselves at least 25 per cent more. Try using large bowls for foods like salad and small ones for ice cream.

Slim secret no. 5
Be Emotionally Slim

Do your emotions send you rushing to the biscuit tin or hiding in a tub of ice cream? After an argument, do you vent your frustration on a bag of crisps?

Well, you're not alone. Many people eat because they're angry, bored, stressed, frustrated, busy or just getting together with friends.

Earlier in the book you learned about the chemical reactions that make you hungry. But often, eating can be triggered by emotions, feelings and thoughts that cause you to wolf down a family-sized packet of biscuits. Experts in the US estimate that as much as 75 per cent of overeating is caused by emotions.

In this chapter you'll learn how your brain and emotions can contribute to your eating behaviour. You'll also gain practical strategies to deal with emotional hunger, dietary traps and everyday situations that make you override your biological satiety signals.

What is emotional hunger?

Emotional hunger means eating when you're not hungry. And it nearly always involves calorie-laden foods such as chocolate, crisps, biscuits and chips instead of healthier foods. An apple just doesn't cut it when you've had a hard day.

How do you distinguish emotional hunger from physical hunger? Well, emotional hunger is urgent and tends to be for a specific food. You might crave chocolate, for example. Nothing else would satisfy. However, if there's no chocolate available, you would eat nothing rather than eat, say, an apple. In other words, you are not genuinely hungry. If you were, you would eat the apple. Emotional hunger also feels uncontrollable, as if something or someone else is putting food in your mouth. And it's nearly always followed by guilt. You hate yourself and vow to make up for your overeating by dieting or exercising.

Food can be used as self-medication to deal with your feelings, problems and stress. Eating can be a way of distracting yourself from getting bored or from facing emotions. German researchers discovered that emotions affect not only the amount people eat but also the type of food they choose and the speed at which they eat. In their study, people ate more when they were angry or happy than when they were fearful or sad. They were more likely to eat quickly and carelessly, or choose foods with strong flavours, when they were angry. They tended to eat to enjoy the taste of food when they felt happy. Interestingly, women were more likely than men to eat quickly when they were angry or sad.

Why do you eat when you're not hungry?

So why, when the going gets tough, do you reach for a chocolate bar?

Your complex relationship with food starts very early in life. From childhood you learn to associate stress reduction with eating and drinking. A baby's blood-sugar level falls if they are hungry. They cry and scream, are fed and feel better. Children are given food when they are upset or sad. They are also offered or denied food as a reward or punishment. So they begin to think of certain foods in terms of comfort, punishment, reward or comfort.

As you move into adulthood and understand more about what's healthy and what's not, the chocolate you were rewarded with as a child becomes a forbidden, guilty indulgence – one you use to reward and compensate yourself with. You might feel that you've earned the right to treat yourself with it after a bad day at work, for example. Your past associations with certain foods means you turn to them when you experience feelings of sadness, anger or happiness.

Eating can be a way of anaesthetising the pain of unmet needs. If your fundamental needs are not met – whether it's for love, comfort, approval, security or control – you turn to food as a replacement.

Chronic stress can also make you eat when you're not really hungry. Scientists at the University of California have found that day-in, day-out stress causes a rise in levels of the stress hormone cortisol, which acts on the part of the brain that controls pleasure-seeking and compulsive behaviours, such as eating, drinking alcohol and taking drugs. For many people, this means seeking solace in comfort food.

Emotional hunger may also be linked to low levels of brain chemicals (such as dopamine, serotonin and endorphins). People who are prone to low levels of serotonin in their brain generally feel better when they eat sugary food. This causes a rise in blood-sugar levels, which in turn causes a rise in levels of serotonin in the brain. And this makes you feel happier.

Can stress make you gain weight?

When you're stressed you release the hormone cortisol. This is part of the 'fight or flight' response, as cortisol release glucose from the body's energy stores to fight or run away. After stress levels have gone down, cortisol hangs around in the bloodstream and stimulates your appetite to make you eat more to replace the energy your body believes you have used up in fighting or running away. The problem is that, nowadays, stress tends to be mental rather than physical. This could be too much work pressure, being stuck in traffic or having a row with your friend. But the body sends out signals to increase your appetite even though it hasn't burned off any extra calories. The result is weight gain. Worse, the fat tends to accumulate around your abdomen as the body stores fat near the liver where it can be converted quickly into fuel ready for the next stressful event. Women are more prone to it than men because they tend to react to events on more of an emotional level.

How to deal with emotional hunger

Facing up to the reasons for overeating isn't easy. There may be a lot of difficult feelings to overcome. The first step is to identify the triggers that make you reach for those comfort snacks. Do you eat when you are bored? Or when you're upset? Or perhaps you take your anger and frustration out on a packet of crisps?

Keep a food and mood diary

Write down everything you eat and drink for a week and jot down how you felt before and after you ate. Soon you'll see a pattern and be able to identify what makes you eat when you're not hungry. Try to pinpoint what it is you need and aren't getting. It might be praise, approval, security, love, success or just a hug.

Find alternatives

Make a list of anything you can think of to help you tackle those feelings without eating. Find outlets for your emotions. For example, if you often eat because you're bored, write down other ways you could occupy yourself. It could be something as simple as going for a walk or a swim. Keep this list handy and, whenever you feel the urge to bury your emotions in food, read through the list.

Deal with your emotions

You don't have to feel angry or upset. If you always do what you've always done, you'll always get what you've always got. The secret is to break out of your comfort zone. Establish new ways of dealing with situations.

De-stress

Emotional eating doesn't actually reduce stress levels. Although you may experience the initial enjoyment of the food in your mouth, your negative feelings don't go away. And if you're stressed, your digestive system finds it harder to process food, leaving you feeling bloated and uncomfortable. The best way to deal with stress is to exercise, so go for a walk or a swim or do some yoga.

Don't buy it

One of the best things you can do is not buy the foods you binge on. Don't bring them into your house, because emotional eating nearly always happens in your own kitchen. If snacks aren't available, you'll automatically find something else to do to change the way you're feeling. Whether it's playing with the kids, housework or reading a book – what these activities have in common is they don't involve food.

Plan ahead

If you know you've got a stressful time coming up, say you're having lots of meetings at work or you're having a difficult time with a partner, plan your food strategy to help you cope better. Plan what healthy meals and snacks you're going to eat and keep all others out of sight.

How to break bad habits

You became overweight through a few bad habits, whether they were snacking on biscuits every time you had a cup of tea or reaching for chocolate every time you felt stressed. The problem with habits is that they are like deep holes: easy to fall into but hard to get out of. Here's how to break those bad habits.

Make a habit list

First you need to identify your bad habits, so make a list of the habits you want to change. This may be: eating crisps while you watch television; having a doughnut with your mid-morning coffee; eating bread with every meal; or eating when you're bored, sad or angry.

Fill your habit holes

Decide how you'll change each habit. Replacing one thing with another is easier than giving something up altogether. Otherwise, when you climb out of that habit hole you'll be left with a gaping hole and you'll probably fall right back in. So aim to fill it with another habit — but this time make it a positive one that helps you feel good and lose weight. You may decide to swap your doughnut for some grapes. But it doesn't necessarily have to be food. You could decide to do something else instead of eating, say, doing the ironing instead of eating while watching TV. Or you may want to break the association with food with a particular location, say by taking your coffee break outside instead of at your desk.

Take one step at a time

Making one change at a time is easier than attempting to make lots of changes. Start with the easiest changes – say, cutting the amount of sugar you take in tea from two teaspoons to one. That way, you won't miss too much. Gradually work up to the tougher or bigger changes.

Here are some ideas for changes you could make:

Old habit	New habit
Snacking in front of the TV	Turn off TV and read a book or go to the gym
Eating biscuits with a cup of tea	Eat an apple
Eating dessert after every meal	Replace with fresh fruit
Nibbling crisps with pre-dinner drinks	Lose the pre-dinner drinks; do something active or go for a walk instead
Mid-morning doughnut at desk	Pop out to buy newspaper/run an errand
Eating big portions	Replace some of main course with extra vegetables

How to avoid dietary pitfalls

However good your eating intentions, you'll find yourself in situations that can jeopardise your weight-loss plans. Whether it's a friend's birthday celebration or shopping in the supermarket, making healthy food choices can be difficult. You don't want to spoil the fun but you also don't want to undo what you've already accomplished. Disruptions to your normal healthy-eating routine will happen and lapses are inevitable. But don't worry – here are some strategies to help you make the best of these tricky situations.

You're not hungry first thing in the morning, so you skip breakfast

The problem: Skipping your morning meal results in low blood-sugar levels by mid-morning, and slows down your metabolism as your body tries to conserve energy until it's fed again. It also slows your thinking and memory recall, according to University of Wales research. As the gap since your last meal grows, you're more likely to slip up mid-morning as you crave sugar and carbohydrates to satisfy your hunger and dipping energy. According to a 2003 study at Harvard Medical School, people who regularly skip breakfast are more likely to overeat later in the day and pile on unwanted pounds.

The quick fix: Whiz up a smoothie with a banana, a pot of low-fat yoghurt and a splash of orange juice to fill you up and boost your blood sugar.

Longer-term solution: Make an effort to streamline your morning schedule so you'll have time to eat breakfast before you go out the door. Get your clothes ready, pack the kids' lunchboxes, make sure they get their school bags packed, and set the breakfast table the night before. No appetite first thing? Then take a wholemeal roll, a pot of yoghurt and couple of satsumas to eat later on (within a couple of hours of waking) and avoid that mid-morning blood-sugar slump.

Your journey to work takes you past the coffee shop and you can't help treating yourself to a takeaway cappuccino and muffin

The problem: Some takeaway coffees can be surprisingly fattening − a cappuccino or latte provides around 200 calories, a large mocha with cream more than 400 calories. Add a blueberry muffin with its 591 calories, and you'll have to adjust your belt − or run 55 minutes at a brisk pace − to burn off that pre-work cappuccino and muffin.

The quick fix: Opt for an espresso (6 calories) or brewed coffee (7 calories). Or go for a 'skinny' cappuccino (calorie save = 46) and skinny muffin (calorie save = 261).

Longer-term solution: Take a different route to work or try swapping your coffee for tea. You'll benefit from tea's antioxidant qualities, which help protect the body from the cell-damaging effects of free radicals. Tea contains polyphenols, which help protect against some cancers and cardiovascular disease. Drinking three cups of tea a day cuts your chances of having a heart attack, say researchers at King's College London, and you can safely drink up to eight cups daily without the risk of caffeine addiction.

You eat lunch late and grab whatever's at hand – not necessarily the healthiest choice

The problem: Eating on the run makes it harder to make slim choices. Fast foods, ready-bought sandwiches and sugary snacks tend to be quick options but are calorie dense so won't help your weight-loss efforts. A hamburger and portion of chips contains 786 calories and 36g fat, a BLT sandwich 540 calories and 26g fat, and a 35g bag of crisps 183 calories and 12g fat.

The quick fix: If you must eat on the run, take a supply of healthy food with you – soup in a flask, pasta salad, a hummus salad roll, fresh fruit, yoghurt – or buy healthier options such as ready-made salads or vegetable soups.

Longer-term solution: Schedule your meals and snacks around your day in advance so you avoid getting too hungry. Plan a healthy snack mid-morning. Try rice cakes with peanut butter, a couple of portions of fruit and a few nuts, or a tuna or cottage-cheese sandwich.

It's someone's birthday (again) and you are expected to partake in the celebratory cake

The problem: A slice of cake can tip your daily calorie balance, ruining your weight-loss efforts. Worse, it can weaken your healthy-eating resolve, and there goes another perfect day.

The quick fix: No one wants to be a party pooper, so accept with good grace but just have half the portion without drawing attention to yourself (or explain: 'I'm not too hungry right now' or 'I've just eaten late lunch').

Longer-term solution: Rather like managing a bank account, allow for the extra calorie load beforehand (e.g. eat one less sandwich for lunch) or later on (e.g. forego dessert at supper). That way your calorie balance need not tip and you have a clear calorie conscience at the end of the day.

You do your supermarket shopping straight after work. You're hungry and there are lots of tempting offers that you can't resist . . .

The problem: When you're hungry, everything edible suddenly becomes tempting, your healthy-eating resolve goes out the window and so you end up buying ready-meals, supersize packs of snacks and two-for-one offers of puds that you wouldn't normally eat.

The quick fix: Never go shopping hungry. Have a small healthy snack (e.g. a slice of toast or an apple) before you go so that cheesecake on special offer won't seem so tempting!

Longer-term solution: Make a list before you go and then buy only what's on the list. Having made your shopping decisions beforehand, you'll have less time to become distracted by special offers. Skip the danger zones by steering a route through the supermarket that avoids the aisles with the cakes, desserts and salty snacks. Cut temptation further by ordering on-line – once you have an established list of 'bought before' foods, your weekly shop can be done in ten minutes.

You've been eating healthily all week and a meal out is your reward. You want everything on the menu, order unhealthy dishes and end up eating too much!

The problem: If you're feeling deprived it's hard to control your desire to make up for it. Over-ordering and overeating is common as the combination of a choice of tempting foods and hunger can prove too much. Any calorie saving made during the week is then cancelled by one meal.

The quick fix: Don't let yourself get too hungry. Have a small protein-rich snack such as a rice cake with peanut butter before you leave for the restaurant so you aren't starving when it's time to order.

Longer-term solution: Plan what to order beforehand. Try to stick, as far as possible, to the amounts and types of food you'd eat at home. Pass on the bread basket before your meal – you wouldn't fill up with bread before your meal at home. Disregard the amount of pasta or pizza you are served – eat your normal portion and leave the rest.

Work colleagues persuade you to go for an after-work drink, against your better judgement

The problem: Alcoholic drinks are high in calories and can tip your daily calorie balance over the edge. A couple of 175ml glasses of wine add 240 'empty' calories to your daily calories. Do this daily and you've swigged 1,680 extra calories in a week, equivalent to half a pound of fat!

The quick fix: Opt for lower-calorie drinks – sparkling water, wine spritzer, low-carb lager, or alternate alcoholic drinks with water or other low-calorie nonalcoholic drinks.

Longer-term solution: Make a calorie adjustment in your day's food intake. Set yourself a limit when you go out and keep a tally on your intake. Do not feel obliged to drink the same amount as your friends – tell them you are driving. Try to eat something first – food slows the absorption of alcohol.

You get home late and hungry without the time, energy or ingredients to rustle up something nutritious and low calorie

The problem: Supper becomes a packet of biscuits eaten in front of the television. When you're ravenous you want to eat the nearest food to hand and that's likely to be calorie-laden snacks.

The quick fix: Keep a supply of healthy snacks for emergencies. Make sure there's always fruit in the fruit bowl, plenty of salad in the fridge, sliced wholemeal bread for toast, and some cartons of yoghurt.

Longer-term solution: Plan ahead – if you know you will be home late, make sure you have healthy standbys in your cupboard so you can make yourself something quick and easy. Add tuna or a tin of beans to pasta sauce and stir into cooked pasta. Try adding chickpeas to ready-made soup.

You suddenly have a craving for something sweet and devour an entire chocolate bar

The problem: Sweets and chocolates are high in calories yet have very poor filling power. A typical chocolate bar contains 250 to 300 calories; a 50g bag of sweets 150 calories. They are easy to overeat because they don't satisfy your hunger.

The quick fix: If you must have something sweet then have your sweet-fix but just a little. A small spoonful of ice cream can feel like a treat. Serve it in a nice bowl and before you sit down to this indulgence, put the tub back in the freezer.

Longer-term solution: Get your sweet fix from naturally sweet foods such as fruit. Grapes, satsumas, pineapples, melons, mangos ... they contain sugar to satisfy your sweet craving but they are also full of fibre and water so they fill you up for relatively few calories. It's harder to overeat fruit than it is to eat a whole packet of sweets or biscuits.

Slim secret no. 6
Get Active

Fitness fads come and go, but the secret to effective weight loss is to combine a programme of regular cardiovascular (aerobic) and strengthening exercise with a balanced diet.

Like most people, you probably think you're fairly active and 'fit enough' for your day-to-day life. But, to lose weight, you need to be active every day – ideally for at least sixty minutes daily, according to national guidelines. This activity should make you breathe faster (though not leave you puffed) and make your heart pump a bit faster. Ideally, you should also include some strengthening (or toning) and stretching activities each week. If that sounds like a tall order, don't worry – it can be broken into several shorter bursts so it fits around your lifestyle, and need not feel as hard as you imagine! The 28-day Eating and Activity Plan (see page 153) shows you how to incorporate all three types of activity into your daily life. The main things to remember are to build up gradually, pick activities you enjoy doing and do them regularly. This chapter will explain how you can get more active and burn fat faster.

Why should I get more active?

Before you begin here are some great reasons for getting active.

Burns fat

Regular activity burns fat, helping you lose weight faster and preventing further weight gain. All movement burns calories – the more you move the more stored fat you'll burn. By losing weight, you'll feel less pain or discomfort in your hips, knees, ankles and back, which will spur you to exercise more.

Benefits your health

Regular activity is good for your health. It halves your risk of developing heart disease, reduces the risk of having a stroke, helps lower blood pressure and reduces the chance of developing diabetes. A study at Harvard University involving 17,000 people found that those who walked 5 to 10 miles a week had a 25 per cent lower risk of heart disease compared to inactive people. It also reduces the risk of several types of cancer (including breast cancer and colon cancer) – Cancer Research UK estimates excess weight causes up to 12,000 cases of cancer a year.

Strengthens your muscles

Doing strength or toning exercises three times a week will prevent the age-related loss of muscle that happens after the age of about thirty. Most people lose between 2.3 and 3.2kg of their muscle every decade, which means a drop in your metabolic rate and daily calorie burn.

Makes your heart stronger

Activity strengthens your heart muscle, allowing it to pump blood efficiently round your body with each heartbeat. Activity also increases the capacity of your lungs so you can breathe in more oxygen with each breath. It also keeps your blood vessels clog-free, helping keep blood cholesterol levels and blood pressure in check.

Lets you live longer

Keeping active means a longer (and healthier) life. In 2003/04, 287,206 people died from diseases associated with a lack of exercise, of which more than 35,000 were directly attributable to physical inactivity.

Relieves stiffness

Stretching exercises relieve stiffness, improve your range of movement and increase your flexibility.

Good for your bones

Weight-bearing exercise, such as walking, running and dancing, slows the bone loss that can lead to osteoporosis (thinning of the bones).

Improves mood and reduces stress

Regular activity can reduce stress, anxiety and depression –
you'll relax more easily and feel better about yourself. It releases
endorphins, chemical messengers that uplift your mood. The Mental
Health Foundation advises that regular moderate exercise can treat
mild to moderate depression as effectively as drugs.

Gives you a good posture

All activities improve your posture, balance, strength, suppleness
and mobility.

Enhances your self-esteem

Regular exercise improves the way you look and makes you feel
better about yourself, so you'll have a greater desire to eat healthily
too.

Gives you more energy

Regular activity makes you feel more energetic. You'll be able to
cope better with your daily routine and have energy to spare.

> Surveys have shown that only 3 or 4 in every 10 men, and 2
> or 3 in every 10 women in the UK are active enough to give
> themselves some protection against heart disease.

How hard should you exercise?

While most leisure activities help to reduce blood pressure and cholesterol levels, some sports, in particular golf or walking, are not vigorous enough to stave off a heart attack, according to a 2007 study at Queen's University Belfast and at Glasgow University. More strenuous activities like jogging, swimming and tennis are better in fighting heart disease. The study found that those who had undertaken vigorous exercise suffered significantly fewer heart attacks than those who had few leisure activities or did light exercise.

Even if you are already active, you can still benefit by adding more activity. The more active you are, the more benefits you will get.

Exercise myths

Myth

Exercising at a low rather than high intensity promotes greater fat loss.

Fact

It is true that the body uses a greater proportion of fats than carbohydrates when exercising at a low intensity. But this doesn't mean that such exercise is better for fat (weight) loss than high-intensity exercise. The most important consideration is the number of calories you burn. During low-intensity exercise the number of fat calories (i.e. the absolute amount of stored fat) will be less than you burn during high-intensity aerobic exercise. The thing to remember is that you lose weight and body fat when you burn more calories than you consume.

Myth

The more you sweat, the more fat you lose.

Fact

When you exercise, especially during hot conditions, you'll certainly sweat and lose weight. But it's mainly lost water, not fat. When you eat or drink next, you'll replenish your body's fluid levels and the lost pounds will return. Sweating is not a good indicator of how many calories you're burning – it simply tells you how much excess heat you are producing and will depend more on the temperature, humidity, the ratio of your weight to surface area and even genetic factors (some people just sweat more).

Myth

You can burn fat from specific regions of your body by exercising those areas.

Fact

Unfortunately you cannot 'spot reduce' fat. When you exercise, you use energy by burning fat from all the regions of the body, not from the specific muscles involved in the exercise. For example, doing abdominal exercises will strengthen your abdominal muscles but won't trim fat off your abdominal area.

Myth

Strength exercises make women bulk up.

Fact

Lots of women are afraid of gaining too much muscle. But lifting weights won't make you bulky. It's one of the quickest and easiest ways for women to look leaner, more sculpted and toned. A pound of muscle takes up a great deal less volume than a pound of fat. It's hard for women to build large muscles as they have low levels of testosterone, a hormone that influences muscle growth.

Myth

Muscle turns to fat when you stop exercising.

Fact

It is impossible for muscle to turn to fat, as it is a completely different type of body tissue. They do not have the capacity to change from one type to another. However, with muscles, it is a case of 'use it or lose it'. If you don't use a muscle it will lose strength, tone and size. If you eat more calories than you burn, the excess will be stored as fat.

Myth

Aerobic exercise stops the loss of lean mass during dieting.

Fact

Aerobic exercise does little to maintain lean mass (muscle) during dieting. The less lean mass you have, the lower will be your metabolic rate. The best way to prevent muscle loss is by combining strength exercises (at least twice a week) with regular aerobic activities.

Simple ways to move your body

First, build more activity into your everyday routine, for example:
- Walk more – look for small ways to walk more: maybe walk to the shops for those small things such as milk or a newspaper, walk your children to school, go for walks with friends, take a walk around the block
- Turn off the TV – try doing something physical instead, like playing games, taking a walk . . . anything active that gets you off the sofa
- Walk up the stairs or escalator instead of using the lift
- Get off the bus a stop earlier and then walk

- Do some chores – working in the garden, raking leaves, doing housework . . . these activities all burn calories
- Put on a CD or tape and dance to it
- Pace while you talk – when you're on the phone pace around and keep moving
- Walk round the block during your lunch break
- Sit on an exercise ball and roll around while you watch TV or work at your desk
- Avoid sitting for long periods – break up sitting periods every thirty minutes (for example, when watching TV get up during adverts or in between programmes)

Next, gradually build up your activity level. Once you have become a little more active, start thinking about which activities you could do regularly. Suitable activities include brisk walking, cycling and dancing.

You may want to involve your partner, family or friends to make it more fun.

How to burn more calories without sweating

A 2005 study conducted by the Mayo Clinic, Rochester, USA, monitored the activity levels of ten lean and ten obese volunteers. What researchers found was that, though neither group did any structured exercise, the lean group burned extra calories just by *moving around more* – no sweating required. The obese volunteers sat for 164 minutes longer each day than the lean group. The lean people were upright for 153 minutes longer than the obese people. The lean group burned an average of 350 extra calories each day (equivalent to 36lb a year) by walking and standing more throughout the day. This proves that the advice you've heard a million times (e.g. take the stairs, walk around more) really does make a difference and can contribute to your weight loss just as much as structured exercise, albeit more slowly.

How much activity?

In 2004, the UK Department of Health announced new exercise guidelines.

To *maintain your health* spend thirty minutes doing moderately intense cardiovascular activity at least five days a week. This means activities that make you breathe faster and your heart beat faster (but not leave you breathless), e.g. brisk walking, gardening, easy-paced swimming, cycling or jogging.

To *prevent weight gain*, you should aim for 45 to 60 minutes moderate cardiovascular exercise a day.

To *lose weight*, you should aim for at least 60 minutes moderate cardiovascular exercise most days of the week.

The American College of Sports Medicine recommends doing activities that burn *at least 2,000 calories* per week.

If that sounds daunting, don't worry – it doesn't have to be done in one go. Several shorter sessions of exercise may actually be better for lowering fat levels in your bloodstream after eating. Researchers from the University of Missouri found that beginners who did ten minutes of exercise at least three times a day had lower blood-fat levels than those who exercised for thirty minutes continuously or did none at all.

How to stay motivated
- Schedule your exercise as if it were an appointment and treat it like one. Write it in your diary and never cancel
- Keep a record of what you did in each workout so you can keep track of your achievements
- Exercise with someone else
- Consider getting a good personal trainer, ideally by word of mouth
- Exercise while wearing clothes that make you feel good and feel comfortable
- Be active to music
- Vary your activity so you don't get bored so, for example, if you normally exercise indoors try an outdoor activity and vice versa

Exercise tips

- *Take it easy to begin with.* Exercise should never feel painful. If you push yourself too hard you risk injuring yourself.
- *Vary your activities.* This will stop you getting bored and make sure that you are exercising your whole body in a balanced way. Most fitness-related injuries are the result of repetitive strain to the same part of the body.
- *Wear comfortable clothes and shoes* that are appropriate for each activity.

- *Pay attention to your breathing.* You should always breathe deeply and regularly. Even when you are working hard, never hold your breath and strain – this will push up your blood pressure and could make you feel dizzy. Try to breathe out as you exert, i.e. on the harder part of a movement.
- *Warm up* each time you do any physical activity – this will help protect your muscles and joints from injury. Five or ten minutes of light exercise that raises your body temperature will do the trick. Begin slowly for the first few minutes and build up gradually.
- *Cool down* when you come to the end of your activity. Take a few minutes to slow down, and make sure you don't stop suddenly. This will help prevent you getting stiff or sore.

How to exercise safely

If you already have a health problem (such as heart disease, asthma, arthritis, diabetes), back problems or if you're not used to doing physical activity, it is important to talk with your GP about the best way to increase your level of physical activity.

It is very important to increase your physical activity gradually. This means both the amount of time you spend doing it, and how intense the activity is.

When not to exercise

- Don't push yourself if you are unwell. It's a myth that you can 'sweat out' a cold.
- Don't exercise if you've got or are recovering from a viral illness

like the flu, if you need to take painkillers to mask pain or if you
have a medical condition and haven't talked to your doctor first.

- Stop exercising if you get any pain in your chest, neck and/or
upper left arm; or if you feel dizzy, sick or unwell, or very tired. If
the symptoms don't go away, or if they come back later, see your
doctor.

Which type of activity?

To achieve a slim and healthy body, you should aim to include
three types of activity in your fitness programme: cardiovascular
exercise, strength (muscle-toning) exercises and stretching. They
are all important for fat loss, though the balance needs to be right.
Cardiovascular activities help burn fat, strength exercises tone your
muscles, and stretching exercises improve flexibility and posture,
making you look slimmer.

Cardiovascular exercise

Cardiovascular (aerobic) activity is any repetitive, rhythmic exercise
involving large muscle groups such as the legs, shoulders and arms.
It increases the body's demand for oxygen and makes the heart and
lungs work harder than usual, making the circulation more efficient,
and helps develop your stamina.

Cardiovascular exercise not only burns calories but also
increases your body's ability to burn fat. Any kind of activity that
uses the large muscle groups of the body and can be kept up
for at least twenty minutes with your heart rate in your target

training range (see page 131) count. Try fast walking, running, cardiovascular training machines, swimming, cycling or group exercise classes. Vary your activities so you don't become too bored. There are two ways of performing cardiovascular activities:

Constant pace

This means you exercise at a steady pace over a longish period. You may work either at a high or low intensity, depending on your fitness level (see box: 'High or low intensity?').

Interval training

Interval training will help you reach your weight loss and fitness goals more quickly. A study at Quebec University found that interval training (90-second bursts at 95 per cent of maximum heart rate) burned three and a half times more body fat than steady-state, moderate-intensity exercise.

Interval training means alternating short bursts of intense activity with lower-intensity periods, during which you recover. Try one or two minutes of high-intensity alternating with two minutes of recovery. If you're swimming, for example, try alternating easy-paced lengths with some fast lengths. Or, if you're walking, experiment by increasing your pace for a few minutes, or running, to get your heart rate up. But don't push yourself too hard, and stop if you feel dizzy, light-headed or sick.

High or low intensity?

Low-intensity activities, such as walking or swimming at an easy pace, burn fat but you will need to do them for longer in order to get the same results. High-intensity cardiovascular activities, such as running or fast swimming, burn more body fat overall because they burn more calories. In a study at the University of Wisconsin, two groups of women were monitored over eight weeks. One group cycled for at a low intensity for 50 minutes daily, the other cycled for just 25 minutes but much more strenuously. At the end of the study all the women lost the same amount of fat. These results show that the higher the intensity of your workout, the quicker you'll burn fat.

Strength exercises

Strength exercises tone your muscles as well as burn stored fat. This doesn't necessarily mean lifting heavy weights – conditioning exercises using your own body weight (such as press-ups or squats) or light weights tone your muscles, and help prevent age-related muscle loss. You won't necessarily burn more calories lifting weights than doing cardiovascular exercise, but the increased muscle mass you develop as a result will make your body burn more calories every day. Every ½kg (1lb) of muscle you add through exercise increases your metabolic rate by 30 to 40 calories a day. That's equivalent to 1,200 extra calories a month, or ½kg (1lb) fat loss in 3 months.

Flexibility

Stretching at the end of each workout will help improve your flexibility and posture, making your muscles look slimmer and longer. It also helps prevent muscle stiffness (especially as you get older), muscle strain and joint injuries. Good flexibility can make a big difference to your posture, appearance and wellbeing. Other fitness activities will feel easier and, if you spend time stretching after exercising, you're less likely to feel sore the next day.

Starting and building an exercise programme

Consistency is the key to fat-burning, so it's important to choose activities that you enjoy and that fit in with your lifestyle. If aerobic classes leave you cold, choose a form of exercise that suits you. It might be walking, tennis, swimming or cycling. If you join a gym, choose one within easy travelling distance of your home or work.

Fitness component	Start with	Once you're fitter
Cardiovascular exercise	Walking, cycling, swimming, aqua aerobics	Aerobic/group exercise classes, running, tennis, hockey, circuit training, kick boxing

Fitness component	Start with	Once you're fitter
Strength exercise	Digging, swimming, hill walking, beginner Pilates classes	Weight training, tubing or resistance bands, circuit training, body-pump classes, Pilates, Ashtanga yoga
Flexibility	Stretch classes, beginner yoga classes	Yoga, tai chi, Pilates

If you're new to exercise, start with low-intensity activities while you build up your fitness. Once you've been exercising for three months, try higher-intensity activities and interval training.

Do early-morning workouts on an empty stomach burn more fat?

If fat loss is your goal, the best time to do cardiovascular exercise is first thing in the morning before eating, when insulin levels are at their lowest and glucagon levels are at their highest. This encourages more fat to leave your fat cells and travel to your muscles, where the fat is burned. You won't necessarily burn more calories, but more of the calories you do burn will come from fat. Over time, this may lead to speedier fat loss.

Work at the right intensity

Make sure you are exercising at a safe and effective level by using one of the following methods:

Talk test

If you can have a leisurely conversation as you exercise, you probably aren't working hard enough. If you can barely gasp a word, slow down!

Heart rate

Take your pulse at your wrist or neck for fifteen seconds. Multiply by four to get the number of beats per minute. Alternatively, use a heart-rate monitor, which will give you a more accurate reading. Most use a chest strap, which relays your heartbeat to a wristwatch device that tells you how fast your heart is beating. Your target during cardiovascular exercise is that your heart should be beating between 60 and 85 per cent of your maximum heart rate (MHR) – see box 'How to calculate your target heart rate'. Working out at between 60 and 70 per cent of MHR will develop everyday fitness and allow you to exercise continuously for at least 20 minutes. Between 70 and 85 per cent MHR develops greater cardiovascular fitness and also burns more fat. Only experienced and serious athletes would exercise at higher heart rates – it is not possible to exercise at this level for long, so use it only as an option for interval training.

Self-perception

You can determine how hard you are working using a 10-point scale, called the Rating of Perceived Exertion (RPE). This ranges from 1 (nothing at all) to 10 (maximum effort) – see box 'RPE' – and correlates well with your heart rate. So aim to exercise at a level that feels fairly hard to you.

How to calculate your target heart rate

The harder you work, the more calories you'll use. As a guide, you should be working at a level at least 60 per cent of your maximum heart rate (MHR). Calculate your MHR by subtracting your age in years from 220. For example, if you are 30 your MHR would be $220 - 30 = 190$ beats per minute. Working out at 60 per cent of this gives $190 \times 0.6 = 114$. But for the fastest improvements in your fitness, try to work nearer to 85 per cent of your MHR.

So, if you are 30, your target heart rate (THR) range would be 114 to 162 beats per minute.

$$THR \text{ (lower limit)} = 190 \times 0.6 = 114$$
$$THR \text{ (upper limit)} = 190 \times 0.85 = 162$$

Working lower than 114 is not efficient for conditioning the heart and lungs or fat-burning, and working higher than 162 will further condition the heart and lungs but will reduce the effectiveness of the fat-burning programme.

Check your heart rate

Age	50% MHR	Target heart rate zone				90% MHR	100% MHR
		60% MHR	70% MHR	80% MHR	85% MHR		
20	100	120	140	160	170	180	200
30	95	114	133	152	162	171	190
40	90	108	126	144	153	162	180
50	85	102	119	136	145	153	170
60	80	96	112	128	136	144	160
70	75	90	105	120	128	135	150
80	70	84	98	112	119	126	140

Rating of perceived exertion (RPE)

Scale level	RPE	Percentage of maximal heart rate	How do you feel?
At rest / light activity – sitting working	1–2	40–55%	Able to talk easily
Light to moderate activity, e.g. walking at leisurely pace	3–4	56–60%	Breathing increases; less easy to talk

Scale level	RPE	Percentage of maximal heart rate	How do you feel?
Moderate activity – brisk walking	5	61–65%	Harder to talk; breathing a little harder; light sweat
Somewhat hard activity – jogging	6	66–70%	Breathing harder
Hard activity – running	7	71–75%	Sweating; breathing harder
Very hard activity – running	8	76–85%	Conversation just possible; sweating heavily
Very, very hard activity – fast running	9	86–95%	Breathing difficult; conversation difficult
Maximum effort – all-out running	10	96–100%	Unable to speak; unable to exercise for very long

Action stations

Ready to go? Take your pick from the activities below and follow the 28-day Eating and Activity Plan (see page 153).

Outdoor activities

Walking is the easiest and cheapest exercise of all – it burns fat if you keep a good pace, pump your arms and walk on an incline whenever possible. It tones your buttocks and all the muscles in your legs and is safer for your back and joints than running.

Walking 4,000 steps a day will benefit your health, 7,000 steps will improve your fitness and 10,000 steps will help you lose weight. You can accumulate these steps throughout the day as you go about your usual activities as well as planned workouts. To find out how many steps you take, attach a pedometer – a simple gadget that measures steps, distance and calories burned – to your belt.

Increase your speed when you no longer feel challenged; reduce the speed if you feel tired. You should feel slightly breathless but comfortable (you should be able to talk in short sentences).

A pair of good shoes is a must. If you intend walking regularly it's worth investing in proper fitness walking shoes. They should feel roomy around the toes, provide good cushioning under the heel, and feel comfortable and light (so your legs don't bear too much extra weight).

Top walking tips:
- Concentrate on keeping a good posture by relaxing your shoulder muscles, keeping your shoulders down (not back), and ribcage slightly lifted.
- Hold your arms relaxed, close to the body, and hands cupped. Avoid swinging your arms across your body.

- As you walk, land on your heel and transfer your weight onto the ball of your foot, rolling the foot in a smooth heel-to-toe movement.
- Stick to a comfortable stride length so your body is not forced to rotate through the hips.
- Keep your hips, knees and feet aligned – your feet should point directly forwards (this may feel awkward at first).
- Keep your body upright or angled just slightly forwards.

Hiking on trails and tracks or up a hill is much more fun than pounding the pavements. It is also a massive calorie burner (up to 500 calories per hour) and the varying terrain improves your fitness quicker than walking on the flat.

Wear several thin layers – comprising modern wicking fabrics such as Cool-Max for maximum coolness – rather than one thicker layer. In hot weather wear loose lightweight clothing that is sweat permeable and light coloured. Do not struggle uphill wearing waterproof clothing.

Take a hat to prevent heat loss in the winter, and to protect your head from the sun and prevent overheating in the summer. Walking boots or shoes with moulded grip-giving soles are a must if the ground is at all hilly or rough. Fitting should be snug but not overtight (you should be able to wiggle your toes without them touching the front of the boot).

Top hiking tips:
- Keep your neck and shoulders relaxed. Look forwards rather than down.

- Keep your arms tucked in close to your body.
- Concentrate power in your back leg and foot as you push off the ground.
- Find a comfortable stride length – keep it short so you won't rotate through the hips.
- Hold your abdominals tight to keep your torso stable and strong.
- Keep your knees and feet aligned – your feet should point directly forwards.

Cycling – get on your bike for a calorie-burning ride. It improves your heart and lungs, burns fat (450 calories per hour), tones the muscles in your thighs, buttocks and lower legs and strengthens the lower back and stomach muscles. Cycling to and from work or the shops integrates exercise into your daily activities, while cycling for fun is a great way to explore the countryside.

Always wear a well-fitting helmet – test this by putting the helmet on and shaking your head. It should not flop around or fall forwards.

If you have knee problems, make sure the seat is high enough and the tension is low – keep in a low gear.

If you have back trouble, avoid bending forwards in the saddle. Cycling on an indoor bike, which is more upright, should relieve the strain.

For maximum fat-burning, aim to maintain a brisk pedalling cadence, between 80 and 110rpm – use lower gears or reduce the tension on an indoor bike. For best muscle tone, use a higher gear or increase the tension. You'll need to drop your pedalling cadence to between 60 and 90rpm.

Off-road cycling requires more upper-body strength and greater balance than road cycling. However, the rewards are a traffic-free environment and more interesting scenery.

Top cycling tips:
- Check your saddle height – in the downward phase of the cycling action, your leg should be extended but bent very slightly at the knee.
- Keep your neck and shoulders relaxed – avoid tensing your shoulders; ensure there is a good distance between your ears and shoulders.
- Keep a neutral spine position in the saddle – keep as upright as possible and don't allow your back to slump forwards.
- Hold your stomach muscles tight – this will help to stabilise you.
- Your toes should point downwards slightly as you push down – this prevents tension in the calf muscles.
- Use toe clips – this allows you to use the muscles at the front and back of your legs to power the movement. Without clips, only the muscles at the front of the legs get worked.

Running is one of the simplest ways to get fit – there's no special equipment or membership fees and, even if you are very busy, you can fit it into your schedule. It tones your thighs, hips, calves and buttocks. A slow run will burn around 175 calories in 20 minutes; a faster pace burns 260 calories.

Make sure that you feel confident with fast walking first – you should be able to walk for 30 minutes easily. Begin with interval running where you run for short periods then fast walk until you recover. Continue to repeat the pattern. Gradually make the running intervals longer and build up the length of your workout. Eventually you'll be able to run for longer periods without needing to stop and walk.

Because running is a high-impact activity, it is not suitable for people with knee problems.

A good pair of running shoes is a must, rather than all-round trainers – they are designed to strike the ground properly, reducing the amount of shock that travels up your leg. They should fit your feet snugly, provide good cushioning on the heel and be flexible enough to allow you to bend your feet naturally.

Top running tips:
- Keep your shoulders back and down in a relaxed comfortable position.
- Use the power in your glutes (buttocks) and hamstrings (back of legs) to propel your body forwards.
- Land on your heels and roll through the whole foot – your toes should be last thing to leave the ground.
- Keep your feet close to the ground and take care not to bounce as you run.
- Keep your arms and hands loose and tension free (don't clench your fists).
- Use a natural backwards and forwards swing with your arms – but don't exaggerate the action.

Skipping is a great form of exercise. It raises your heart rate and your spirits and can bring back the joys of childhood into your life. All you need is a skipping rope and a tall enough ceiling and space to turn the rope without knocking over a lamp or whipping your dog's tail. Skipping at a moderate speed (70 to 120 turns per minute) for 15 minutes burns 150 to 200 calories.

It's great for developing your balance, co-ordination, rhythm and timing, and strengthens your legs, shoulders and arms.

Alternating feet when skipping is easy to learn: aim to jump a few times on one foot, and then try the other foot. Soon you will be able to go from one to the other without catching the rope.

Whilst skipping, the rope should ideally be tight, and if jumping at speed, aim to have small jumps, with the rope close to your head.

Skipping to music, using different foot combinations and also adding circuit exercises will prevent you becoming bored.

Start with short, 15- to 20-second bouts of skipping interspersed with 30 to 40 seconds of complete rest or light marching on the spot. Repeat this pattern five to ten times. As your stamina increases, lengthen your skipping bouts and shorten your rests.

Once you can skip for at least five minutes straight, mix up your footwork. Try hopping on one foot then the other at each turn, or alternately landing on the heel of one foot and then on the ball of the other.

Top skipping tips:
- Jump just enough to clear the rope – any higher can put strain on your knees.
- Aim for an easy transfer of body weight from one foot to the other as you skip.

- Land with knees slightly bent.
- Keep your back straight, with your shoulders relaxed and down.
- Aim to keep your elbows tucked into your sides, at waist level, with the rope turning around smoothly in your wrists.
- A common mistake is to lean forwards, or skip too slowly. Both of these result in the rope being caught by your feet.

Swimming gives a great all-round workout. It tones all of the major muscles in the body and is kinder to your joints and back than land training. If you are new to exercise or are prone to back problems, it's a particularly effective way of getting fit. It burns between 240 and 300 calories per 30 minutes. It is good for maintaining flexibility, especially around the shoulders

If you are new to swimming, use a float to provide buoyancy. Hold it in front of you with both hands as you kick your legs. Intersperse water walking with length swimming to increase your total exercise time.

Water can feel relaxing but if you are trying to improve your fitness you will need to push yourself. You should not be able to talk comfortably – just one-word answers if pushed!

Top swimming tips (front crawl):
- For a really effective workout it's best to use stronger strokes such as the front crawl.
- Turn your head to the side to breathe in, bringing your ear close to your shoulder rather than lifting your head out of the water.
- Reach directly in front of you. Keep your hand slightly cupped as you pull through the stroke.

- Pull through the central line of the body, keeping the arm slightly bent.
- Kick from the hip, using the entire leg, not just the lower portion.
- Concentrate on keeping your hips level and aim to minimise rotation of your body.

In the gym

A gym or health club is a good environment for exercising without distractions. Use the exercise bike, treadmill, rowing machine, elliptical trainer or stairclimber. The first time you go on the machine, ask a fitness instructor to show you how the machine works.

Most machines indicate the calories burned, which helps gauge your progress, but the readouts may not be accurate for everyone. Focus instead on distance covered, intensity or duration of your workouts.

Rowing is excellent for all-round fitness, working all the major muscles at the same time. The indoor rowers found in most gyms provide a good simulation of the real thing, without getting your feet wet. You can burn 50 to 150 calories in 10 minutes depending on the resistance and speed.

Top rowing tips:
- Use the foot straps to keep your feet firmly in the machine, and keep your bottom firmly on the seat.
- Use your leg muscles to power the movement. Start the stroke by pushing with your legs to drive you back along the machine — don't pull with your arms.

- Keep your arms extended in front of you until they reach the knees, then lean back slightly, pulling the handle towards your body.
- Bring the handle into your abdomen not to your chest. Your elbows should be drawn past the body, not sticking out.
- At the end of the stroke, take care not to 'lock' your legs straight – keep the knees soft.
- Don't go for speed at the expense of technique. Aim to keep a smooth motion throughout, with a stroke rate (how many times you go back and forth) at around 26 to 33 strokes per minute.

The treadmill is a great alternative to walking or running outdoors. It offers more shock absorption, which makes it easier on your joints, and it lets you work out whatever the weather. You can walk, jog and run and you can even climb hills by adjusting the gradient. A slow jog (5mph) burns 200 calories in 20 minutes; a brisk run (10mph) burns 400 calories.

Try to use a natural stride length and power the movement from your buttocks and hamstrings. Using too short strides will stress your knees.

If you have knee or back problems, walk rather than run.

To start with, select a programme that allows you to talk fairly easily. As you get used to the machine, increase the speed and/or gradient – you should feel slightly out of breath but talking should be just possible.

Working out on a treadmill is slightly easier than doing the same activity outside because there's no wind resistance. To counteract this, you should set the treadmill on an incline of 1 or 2 per cent.

Top treadmill tips:

- The secret is not to panic the first time you go on the treadmill.
- Start with walking to build up your confidence and fitness. Then, when you get used to the machine, you can increase the speed.
- Drop your shoulders and keep them relaxed.
- Keep your eyes in front until you feel more confident.
- Swing your arms easily by your sides.
- Allow your heel to land first and roll forward before pushing off with your toes.
- Your feet, knees and hips should be in good alignment.
- Maintain an upright posture and keep your spine in neutral position.

The elliptical trainer (also called the cross-trainer) provides a no-impact alternative to running on the treadmill, and also targets a wider range of muscles. The machine takes your legs through an elliptical motion that is a cross between running, stepping and cross-country skiing, so you get the benefits of all these exercises. It burns between 180 and 300 calories per 20 minutes, depending on the resistance and speed.

To start with, select a resistance level (around 5 to 7) or inbuilt workout programme that allows you to talk fairly easily. As you get used to the machine, increase the resistance — you should feel slightly out of breath but talking should be just possible. As you get fitter, you can increase your workout time and add high-intensity intervals.

Top elliptical training tips:

- Maintain a good upright posture.
- Keep your shoulders back and relaxed.

- Look forwards, not down at your feet – your head should be level.
- Make sure your weight is evenly distributed and that your lower body supports most of your weight.
- Relax and maintain a comfortable smooth stride going through the normal range of motion.
- Avoid leaning too far forwards and hunching over the handles (which can be stressful for the back).

Toning exercises

These will help tone and strengthen specific muscles. Start with ten repetitions and add two reps once you can complete ten easily. Use the full range of motion, taking the muscle from its fully extended position to its fully contracted position. For exercises with weights, select a weight that allows you to complete ten to fifteen reps with good control. Increase the weight once you can complete fifteen reps easily. Maintain good posture and neutral alignment of your spine throughout each exercise.

Which level are you?

Level 1 (beginner) – You haven't done any serious exercise for at least a year. Just follow the basic instructions for each exercise.

Level 2 (intermediate) – You exercise about once a week and lead quite an active lifestyle. Try the additional options as specified.

Level 3 (advanced) – You exercise regularly (at least two or three times a week). Try the additional options as specified.

Free-standing squat

Great for: Toned legs and bottom.

Basic: Stand with your feet shoulder-width apart, toes angled out at 30 degrees. With your arms held out in front of you, slowly lower yourself down until your thighs are parallel to the ground. Keep your knees aligned over your feet, pointing in the direction of your toes. Hold for a count of one, then return to the starting position. You should maintain the natural curve in your back throughout the movement. Make sure you do not bend forwards excessively as this will stress your lower back and reduce the emphasis on your legs. Do ten to fifteen repetitions.

Level 2 and 3: Make it harder by holding a pair of dumbbells by your sides.

Lunges

Great for: Lifting the bottom.

Basic: Stand with your feet shoulder-width apart, toes pointing forwards. Take a large step backwards with your right leg, as you bend your left leg and lower your hips. Keep your trunk upright.

Lower yourself into a one-legged squat position on your left leg until your left thigh is parallel to the floor. Your left knee should be at an angle of 90 degrees. Hold for a second, then push hard through your left leg to return to the starting position. Don't push through your right (back) leg. Repeat for ten to fifteen reps, then repeat with the left leg leading.

Keep your body erect throughout the movement – do not lean forwards.

Level 2 and 3: Make it harder by holding a pair of dumbbells by your sides.

Press-ups

Great for: Shaping the chest and arms.

Basic: Kneel on the floor with your knees directly under your hips. Place your hands slightly wider than shoulder-width apart under your shoulders, fingers pointing forwards. Keeping a straight line through your torso, bend your arms until your nose almost touches the floor. Aim your chest between your hands. Straighten your arms back to the start position. Repeat for ten to fifteen reps.

Level 2: Do extended press-ups; this time make a straight line from your knees to head and raise your lower legs to 90 degrees.

Level 3: Do full press-ups keeping you legs and body straight and feet hip-width apart.

Crunches

Great for: A toned tummy.

Basic: Lie flat on your back on the floor with your knees bent over your hips and your ankles touching. Place your hands lightly by the sides of your head or across your chest. Press your lower back to the floor and use your abdominal strength to raise your head and shoulders from the floor. You should only come up about 10cm and your lower back should remain on the floor. Hold this position for a moment then let your body uncurl slowly back to the starting position. Do ten to fifteen repetitions.

Level 2: Fifteen to twenty repetitions.

Level 3: Twenty to twenty-five repetitions.

Plank

Great for: A flat tummy.

Basic: Lie face down on the floor with your hips and legs in contact with the floor, your upper body raised and supported on your forearms. Your elbows should be directly under your shoulders by the sides of your body, palms down.

Lift your hips so that only your forearms and toes are on the floor. Keep your spine in neutral alignment – your head, back, hips and ankles should be in a straight line. Hold for ten to fifteen seconds and then slowly lower back to the start position.

Level 2: Hold for thirty seconds.

Level 3: Hold for forty-five to sixty seconds.

Shoulder press

Great for: Shapely shoulders.

Basic: Sit on the edge of a bench or an exercise ball. Hold a pair of dumbbells, hands facing forwards, level with your shoulders. Press the dumbbells upwards and inwards until they almost touch over your head. Straighten your arms but do not lock out your elbows. Hold for a count of one. Lower the dumbbells slowly back to the starting position and repeat for ten to fifteen reps.

Level 2 and 3: Use a heavier weight.

Triceps dip

Great for: Toned arms.

Basic: Use a sturdy bench or chair for this exercise. Place your hands shoulder-width apart, fingers facing forwards, on the edge of the bench. Place your feet hip-width apart. Keeping your back straight and close to the bench, bend your elbows and lower your body until your elbows make an angle of 90 degrees. Straighten your arms to bring you back to the starting position. Do ten to fifteen repetitions.

Level 2 and 3: Place your heels on another bench so that your legs form a straight bridge between the two benches.

Back extension

Great for: Strengthening the lower back.

Basic: Lie face down on the floor. Place your arms behind your back. Slowly raise your head, shoulders and upper chest from the floor. This will be just a short distance. Pause for a count of two; then lower slowly to the floor. Keep your head facing downwards to the floor in line with your spine. Do ten to fifteen repetitions.

Level 2 and 3: Place your hands by the sides of your head, elbows out to the sides.

One-arm dumbbell row

Great for: Shaping the upper back and good posture.

Basic: Hold a dumbbell in your right hand, palm facing your body. Bend forwards from the hips, placing your left hand and knee on a bench to stabilise yourself. Your back should be flat and almost horizontal and your right arm fully extended. Pull the dumbbell up towards your waist, drawing your elbow back as far as it can go. Keep the dumbbell close to your body. Allow the dumbbell to touch your ribcage lightly. Pause for a count of one; then slowly lower the dumbbell until your arm is fully extended. Repeat for ten to fifteen reps then perform the exercise with your left arm.

Level 2 and 3: Use a heavier weight.

Stretching exercises

You should only stretch when your body is warm. Stretching a cold muscle increases the risk of injury and reduces the effectiveness of the stretch. Make sure you listen to your body and ease out of the stretch if you feel any pain. Here are some guidelines:

- Gradually ease into position, focusing all the time on relaxing the muscle.
- Stretch only as far as is comfortable and then hold that position. As the muscle relaxes ease further into the stretch, gradually increasing the range of movement.
- Don't bounce or force a movement.
- Exhale and relax as you go into the stretch and then breathe normally.
- Never go past the point of discomfort or pain. You could pull or tear the muscle or tendon.
- Stretches should be held for fifteen to thirty seconds (or longer if you have time).
- Release from the stretch slowly.

Front thigh stretch

Hold on to a sturdy support. Bend one leg behind you and hold your ankle. Keeping your thighs level and knees close together, push your hips forwards until you feel a good stretch. Repeat on the other side.

Hamstring stretch

Sit on the floor with one leg extended and the other leg bent. Keeping your back straight and flat, hinge forwards from the hips. Reach down towards your foot. Flexing your foot will increase the stretch on the calf. Repeat on the other side.

Calf stretch

From a standing position, take an exaggerated step forwards, keeping your rear leg straight. Hold on to a wall for support if you wish. Your front knee should be at 90 degrees and positioned over your foot. Lean forwards slightly so that your rear leg and body make a continuous line. Repeat with the other leg.

Lower back stretch

Lie on your back, knees bent and arms straight out to each side. Rotate both legs to each side, keeping your head, shoulders and arms in contact with the floor.

Upper back stretch

Clasp your hands together and push your arms straight out in front of you at shoulder level so that you feel a good stretch between your shoulder blades.

Shoulder stretch

Bring one arm across your body at shoulder height, aiming the elbow towards the opposite shoulder. Place the opposite hand on the upper arm and press gently until you feel a good stretch in your shoulder. Repeat on the other side.

Chest and arm stretch

With your arm fully extended, hold on to an upright support at shoulder level. Gently turn your body away from your arm, pressing your shoulder forwards. Repeat on the other side.

The 28-day Eating and Activity Plan

After reading the previous six chapters you may have started to make a few changes to the way you eat and the amount of activity you do. Perhaps, by now, you have started to unravel some of the reasons behind your old eating habits; you may be viewing your relationship with food more positively and are now feeling a little more in control. That's a great start. Maybe you've begun to eat more satiating foods, added more vegetables to your meals, changed one or two unhealthy habits to more healthy ones, or are just more aware of portion sizes of the foods you normally eat. Perhaps you've already upped your daily activity or even tried something new.

Or you could be wondering exactly how and where to begin. Putting lots of new information into practice can seem daunting. Especially when there may be so many things that you'd like to change.

Don't worry – this 28-day Eating and Activity Plan will set you on the path to healthy habits. It combines the eating and activity advice contained in the first six chapters of this book. Think of it as a blueprint for your future eating and exercising habits. You can follow part of it or all of it, or even repeat it as often as you want.

It comprises a day-by-day eating plan and activity plan. The daily menus are interchangeable, so if you want to swap meals between different days you can. You can even repeat daily menus if you find they fit particularly well into your daily schedule. But you should stick to the activity plan given for each day as this is designed to build up over 28 days — the idea is that you progressively increase the number of times per week, the amount of time and also the intensity of your activity.

In the eating plan:
- Exact portion sizes are not given for most foods in the plan because everyone needs slightly different amounts of foods (and calories). I give a guide to portion sizes only for calorie-dense foods, such as cheese, nuts and meat, where it's important to keep a tighter rein on the amount you eat.
- Try to be guided by your own appetite and calorie needs. The more active you are, the more food (and calories) you need.
- No food is banned. Simply balance your diet by eating smaller amounts — and less often — of those foods with a high calorie density, and larger amounts of foods with a low calorie density. Don't cut out 'healthy' calorie-dense foods like cheese, nuts and olive oil, because they supply important nutrients that would be hard to get from other foods.
- Be generous with low-calorie foods, such as vegetables, fruit, vegetable dishes and low-fat dairy foods. Fill your plate with

vegetables, and enjoy large portions of dishes like vegetable soup, salad and fresh fruit.

- Plan your weekly menu so you can organise shopping at least a few days ahead and ensure you have all the ingredients to hand.

The activity plan consists of three sections:

1. Cardiovascular activity to help you burn fat and lose weight.
2. Strength/toning exercises – to tone and sculpt your body, improve posture and help strengthen your bones.
3. Stretching – to reduce the likelihood of soreness as well increase your flexibility.

You should do all three types of activity as specified. Each one produces unique benefits – don't be tempted to skip any of them (although some days are rest days, and on other days you will only need to perform one or two of the three parts).

For all levels, spend ten minutes warming up doing light cardiovascular exercise (e.g. brisk walking, slow jogging, or on an exercise machine). Begin slowly for the first few minutes and build up gradually. You should feel warm and just break into a light sweat.

Which level are you?

Level 1 (beginner) – You haven't done any serious exercise for at least a year.

Level 2 (intermediate) – You exercise about once a week and lead quite an active lifestyle.

> Level 3 (advanced) You exercise regularly (at least two or
> three times a week).

WEEK 1

Day 1

Eating plan

Breakfast　Porridge (page 203) *or* 1 slice of wholemeal toast with
honey and fresh fruit

Lunch　Spicy couscous salad (page 206) *or* jacket potato with
baked beans and salad

Supper　Roasted winter vegetable ratatouille (page 219) *or*
chicken salad with whole-grain rice
Fresh fruit for dessert

Snacks　Satsuma and grapes; small handful (25g) of nuts

Drink　At least 8 glasses or cups (1½ litres) of water, herbal or
fruit tea, ordinary tea or green tea. (You may also include up to
2 cups of coffee without sugar if you wish.)

Activity plan

Cardiovascular activity: Choose any of the cardiovascular
activities listed on pages 134–44. Perform your workout at a
constant pace at a moderate intensity (RPE 5, or 60 to 65 per cent
MHR). It should make you breathe a little harder and break into a
light sweat by the end.

Level 1: 20 minutes

Level 2: 25 minutes
Level 3: 30 minutes

Strength/toning: Do the toning exercises described on pages 144–50. Perform the number of repetitions indicated for your fitness level. Rest for 30 seconds between each exercise. Make sure you focus on your form and technique.

Stretching: After the toning exercises, perform the stretches described on pages 150–2. Hold each stretch for 30 seconds.

Day 2

Eating plan

Breakfast   Strawberry banana smoothie (page 201) *or* fresh fruit and a pot of yoghurt

Lunch   Moroccan-style lentil soup (page 207) with 1 slice of whole-grain bread *or* large salad with tuna or beans

Supper   Vegetable balti with chickpeas (page 220) *or* baked potato (see 'The perfect baked potato', page 214) with grilled white fish and vegetables

Snacks   2 plums; 10 strawberries; 1 pot low-fat yoghurt

Drink   At least 8 glasses or cups (1½ litres) of water, herbal or fruit tea, ordinary tea or green tea. (You may also include up to 2 cups of coffee without sugar if you wish.)

Activity plan

Rest day

Day 3

Eating plan

Breakfast   1 breakfast muffin (page 203) with a banana *or* 1 slice
of wholemeal toast and honey with fresh fruit

Lunch   Rocket and courgette frittata with warm tomato sauce
(page 208) with salad *or* Avocado and tomato salad

Supper   Grilled coconut fish (page 221) *or* fish of your choice
with new potatoes, broccoli and green beans
Apple sorbet (page 233) *or* 1 scoop of sorbet of your choice

Snacks   Pear, kiwi fruit and a small handful (25g) of nuts

Drink   At least 8 glasses or cups (1½ litres) of water, herbal or
fruit tea, ordinary tea or green tea. (You may also include up to
2 cups of coffee without sugar if you wish.)

Activity plan

Cardiovascular activity: Try to pick a different cardiovascular activity
today. Again, perform your workout at a constant pace at a moderate
intensity (RPE 5, or 60 to 65 per cent MHR). It should make you
breathe a little harder and break into a light sweat by the end.

Level 1: 20 minutes
Level 2: 25 minutes
Level 3: 30 minutes

Day 4

Eating plan

Breakfast   1 slice wholemeal toast with honey with 1 pot of low-
fat yoghurt and fresh fruit

Lunch   Vegetable soup (page 207) *or* 250ml ready-bought
vegetable soup with 1 wholemeal roll
  Fresh fruit of your choice

Supper   Chicken roasted with butternut squash (page 221),
broccoli and a baked potato *or* grilled chicken breast with
steamed vegetables and a baked potato

Snacks   85g fresh berries, 2 satsumas and 25g (size of 4 dice)
cheese

Drink   At least 8 glasses or cups (1½ litres) of water, herbal or
fruit tea, ordinary tea or green tea. (You may also include up to
2 cups of coffee without sugar if you wish.)

Activity plan

Rest day

Day 5

Eating plan

Breakfast   Fruit muesli (page 204) with skimmed milk *or* bran
flakes with skimmed milk and fresh fruit

Lunch   Roasted herby tomato salad (page 210) with 1 slice
wholemeal bread *or* large leafy salad with a small turkey breast
and 1 slice wholemeal bread

Supper   Trout with roasted Mediterranean vegetables (page 222)
and a baked potato *or* grilled oily fish with steamed vegetables
and a baked potato
  Fresh fruit salad

Snacks   1 slice of melon, 1 apple and 1 pot of low-fat yoghurt
Drink   At least 8 glasses or cups (1½ litres) of water, herbal or
fruit tea, ordinary tea or green tea. (You may also include up to
2 cups of coffee without sugar if you wish.)

Activity plan

Cardiovascular activity: Choose one of the cardiovascular
activities listed on pages 134–44. Perform your workout at a
constant pace but, today, try to step up your pace a little, aiming
for a moderate to hard intensity (RPE 5 to 6, or 60 to 70 per cent
MHR). It should make you breathe a little harder than before and
break into a light sweat by the end.

Level 1: 25 minutes
Level 2: 30 minutes
Level 3: 35 minutes

Strength/toning: Do the toning exercises described on pages
144–50. Perform the number of repetitions indicated for your
fitness level. Rest for 30 seconds between each exercise. Make
sure you focus on your form and technique.

Stretching: After the toning exercises, perform the stretches
described on pages 150–2. Hold each stretch for 30 seconds.

Day 6

Eating plan

Breakfast   Tropical smoothie (page 201) *or* fresh fruit and 1 pot
of low-fat yoghurt

Lunch Asparagus and broad bean salad with poached egg (page 211) and 1 slice wholemeal bread *or* wholemeal hummus sandwich with large salad

Supper Baked red peppers with lentils and goats' cheese (page 223), carrots and new potatoes *or* baked potato with baked beans, carrots and sweetcorn

Raspberry and Passion Fruit Fool (page 234) or 1 pot low-fat fruit yoghurt

Snacks 1 banana and a small handful (25g) of nuts or seeds

Drink At least 8 glasses or cups (1½ litres) of water, herbal or fruit tea, ordinary tea or green tea. (You may also include up to 2 cups of coffee without sugar if you wish.)

Activity plan

Rest day

Day 7

Eating plan

Breakfast Yoghurt with dried fruit compote (page 204) or fresh fruit with 1 pot of yoghurt

Lunch Salmon and bean salad (page 212) *or* wholemeal salmon sandwich with salad

Fresh fruit of your choice

Supper Pasta with chickpeas and spinach (page 224) *or* mixed bean salad with 1 wholemeal roll

Snacks 2 apricots, a small bowl (85g) of berries, 25g (size of 4 dice) cheese

Drink   At least 8 glasses or cups (1½ litres) of water, herbal or
fruit tea, ordinary tea or green tea. (You may also include up to
2 cups of coffee without sugar if you wish.)

Activity plan

Cardiovascular activity: This is a repeat of Day 5. Perform your
workout at a constant pace, aiming for a moderate to hard intensity
(RPE 5 to 6, or 60 to 70 per cent MHR). It should make you breathe
a little harder than before and break into a light sweat by the end.

Level 1: 25 minutes
Level 2: 30 minutes
Level 3: 35 minutes

Stretching: After the cardiovascular activity, perform the stretches
described on pages 150–2. Hold each stretch for 30 seconds.

WEEK 2

Day 8

Eating plan

Breakfast   Fresh fruit salad with honey (page 205) *or* Strawberry
banana smoothie (page 201)

Lunch   Asian prawn salad (page 212) with 1 slice wholemeal
bread *or* a baked potato with prawns and salad

Supper   Vegetable stir-fry with sesame noodles (page 224) *or*
steamed vegetables of your choice with whole-grain rice and a
small handful of nuts or seeds

Snacks   10 strawberries, 1 pear and 1 pot of low-fat yoghurt
Drink   At least 8 glasses or cups (1½ litres) of water, herbal or
fruit tea, ordinary tea or green tea. (You may also include up to
2 cups of coffee without sugar if you wish.)

Activity plan

Rest day

Day 9

Eating plan

Breakfast   Porridge (page 203) or 1 small bowl of whole-grain
breakfast cereal with 1 tbsp of dried fruit and skimmed milk
Lunch   Chicken and lentil salad (page 213) *or* ready-bought lentil
soup with a small wholemeal roll
Fresh fruit of your choice
Supper   Moroccan vegetable tagine (page 225) *or* couscous
mixed with vegetables and chickpeas
Spiced fruit skewers (page 235) or fresh fruit
Snacks   1 pot of low-fat yoghurt and 1 apple
Drink   At least 8 glasses or cups (1½ litres) of water, herbal or
fruit tea, ordinary tea or green tea. (You may also include up to
2 cups of coffee without sugar if you wish.)

Activity plan

Cardiovascular activity: Try to choose a different cardiovascular
activity today, if possible. Perform your workout at a constant pace,
but try to push yourself a little harder today. Aim for RPE 6, or 65

to 70 per cent MHR. It should make you breathe a little harder than
before and break into a moderate sweat by the end.

    Level 1: 30 minutes

    Level 2: 35 minutes

    Level 3: 40 minutes

Strength/toning: Do the toning exercises described on pages
144–50. Perform the number of repetitions indicated for your
fitness level. Rest for 30 seconds between each exercise, then
repeat, so you perform the whole sequence twice. Level 2 and Level
3 exercisers should increase the weight or reps a little.

Stretching: After the toning exercises, perform the stretches
described on pages 150–2. Hold each stretch for 30 seconds.

Day 10

Eating plan

Breakfast 1 slice wholemeal toast with a poached egg *or* 1 small
    bowl of whole-grain cereal with skimmed milk

Lunch A baked potato with hummus or ratatouille or other filling
    suggestion on page 214

    Fresh fruit of your choice

Supper Lentil and red pepper dahl (page 226) with whole-grain
    rice *or* a mixed bean salad with a baked potato

Snacks A small handful (25g) of nuts and dried fruit (25g); 1
    satsuma

Drink At least 8 glasses or cups (1½ litres) of water, herbal or

fruit tea, ordinary tea or green tea. (You may also include up to 2 cups of coffee without sugar if you wish.)

Activity plan

Rest day

Day 11

Eating plan

Breakfast   Blueberry smoothie (page 202) or a small bowl (85g) of berries with a pot of low-fat yoghurt

Lunch   Tuna and white bean salad (page 215) *or* a baked potato with baked beans and a little grated cheese
Fresh fruit of your choice

Supper   Sweet-and-sour chicken with mango (page 227) with basmati rice *or* chicken and rice salad with vegetables

Snacks   2 kiwi fruit and 1 banana

Drink   At least 8 glasses or cups (1½ litres) of water, herbal or fruit tea, ordinary tea or green tea. (You may also include up to 2 cups of coffee without sugar if you wish.)

Activity plan

Cardiovascular activity: Today is a repeat of Day 9. Aim for RPE 6, or 65 to 70 per cent MHR. It should make you breathe a little harder than before and break into a moderate sweat by the end.
Level 1: 30 minutes
Level 2: 35 minutes
Level 3: 40 minutes

Stretching: After the cardiovascular activity, perform the stretches described on pages 150–2. Hold each stretch for 30 seconds.

Day 12

Eating plan

Breakfast   Yoghurt with dried fruit compote (page 204) *or* fresh fruit with 1 pot of low-fat yoghurt

Lunch   Pitta pockets (page 215) *or* a wholemeal roll with chicken and salad

Fresh fruit of your choice

Supper   Fish with spicy chickpeas (page 228) with carrots *or* a leafy salad with mixed beans

Exotic fruit salad (page 235)

Snacks   A small handful (25g) of nuts and a banana

Drink   At least 8 glasses or cups (1½ litres) of water, herbal or fruit tea, ordinary tea or green tea. (You may also include up to 2 cups of coffee without sugar if you wish.)

Activity plan

Cardiovascular activity: Perform your workout at a constant pace. You should try to push yourself a bit harder than yesterday. Aim for RPE 7, or 70 to 75 per cent MHR. It should make you breathe a little harder than before and sweat a little more than before!

Level 1: 35 minutes
Level 2: 40 minutes
Level 3: 45 minutes

Strength/ toning: This is the same as Day 9's workout. Do the toning sequence twice.

Stretching: After the toning exercises, perform the stretches described on pages 150–2. Hold each stretch for 30 seconds.

Day 13

Eating plan

Breakfast   Cranberry orange smoothie (page 202) *or* porridge (page 203)

Lunch   Turkey and avocado sandwich (page 216) *or* leafy salad with hummus
Fresh fruit of your choice

Supper   Tarragon chicken breasts on lentils and mushrooms (page 229) *or* lentil salad with a baked potato
Apple sorbet (page 233) or fresh fruit

Snacks   A small bunch of grapes, an apple and 25g (size of 4 dice) of cheese

Drink   At least 8 glasses or cups (1½ litres) of water, herbal or fruit tea, ordinary tea or green tea. (You may also include up to 2 cups of coffee without sugar if you wish.)

Activity plan

Rest day

Day 14

Eating plan

Breakfast Breakfast muffin (page 203) with fresh fruit *or* 1 slice of wholemeal toast with honey and fresh fruit

Lunch Hummus with vegetable sticks (page 217) and a small wholemeal pitta *or* vegetable soup with a small wholemeal roll

Supper Roast vegetable and bean lasagne (page 230) *or* a baked potato with roast vegetables and a small grilled fish fillet

Snacks 1 small bowl (85g) of berries, 1 apple and a small handful (25g) of nuts or seeds

Drink At least 8 glasses or cups (1½ litres) of water, herbal or fruit tea, ordinary tea or green tea. (You may also include up to 2 cups of coffee without sugar if you wish.)

Activity plan

Cardiovascular activity: This is a repeat of Day 12 but try to do a different cardiovascular activity today to give your body a new challenge. Aim for RPE 7, or 70 to 75 per cent MHR. It should make you breathe a little harder than before and sweat a little more than before!

> Level 1: 35 minutes
> Level 2: 40 minutes
> Level 3: 45 minutes

Strength/toning: Reduce the rest time between exercises to 20 seconds and repeat the toning sequence twice.

Stretching: After the toning exercises, perform the stretches described on pages 150–2. Hold each stretch for 30 seconds.

WEEK 3

Day 15

Eating plan

Breakfast   Porridge (page 203) *or* 1 small bowl of whole-grain cereal with skimmed milk and fresh fruit

Lunch   Butternut squash soup with cannellini beans (page 218) with 1 slice of wholemeal bread *or* a rice and bean salad with tomatoes

Fresh fruit of your choice

Supper   Puy lentils with Mediterranean vegetables (page 231) with a baked potato and leafy salad *or* a lentil and vegetable casserole

Roasted peaches and plums with yoghurt (page 236) *or* fresh peaches

Snacks   2 rice cakes with peanut butter and 1 orange

Drink   At least 8 glasses or cups (1½ litres) of water, herbal or fruit tea, ordinary tea or green tea. (You may also include up to 2 cups of coffee without sugar if you wish.)

Activity plan

Cardiovascular activity: Today you'll do an interval workout, alternating short bursts of intense activity with lower-intensity periods. After your warm-up do one minute at a faster pace, then one minute at a slower pace. Repeat. If you're swimming, for example, alternate one or two easy-paced lengths with fast lengths. Or, if you're walking, alternate one minute fast walking with one minute running. Aim to work at RPE 8, or 75 to 85 per cent MHR during the high-intensity intervals.

Level 1: Repeat 10 times
Level 2: Repeat 12 times
Level 3: Repeat 15 times

Strength/toning: Today, you'll perform two 'sets' of each exercise. Perform the number of reps for your fitness level, rest for 30 seconds, then repeat. Rest again for 30 seconds and move on to the next exercise. Again, perform this exercise twice and do the same with the other exercises.

Stretching: After the toning exercises, perform the stretches described on pages 150–2. Hold each stretch for 30 seconds.

Day 16

Eating plan

Breakfast   1 tropical smoothie (page 201) *or* a bowl of fresh fruit with low-fat yoghurt

Lunch   Spicy couscous salad (page 206) *or* a pasta salad with tuna

Fresh fruit of your choice

Supper   Chicken soup (page 232) with a wholemeal roll *or* a large salad with mixed beans

Snacks   2 plums and 1 pot of low-fat yoghurt

Drink   At least 8 glasses or cups (1½ litres) of water, herbal or
fruit tea, ordinary tea or green tea. (You may also include up to
2 cups of coffee without sugar if you wish.)

Activity plan

Rest day

Day 17

Eating plan

Breakfast   Fruit muesli (page 204) *or* 1 slice of wholemeal toast
with honey and 1 pot of low-fat yoghurt

Lunch   Moroccan-style lentil soup (page 207) *or* baked beans on
wholemeal toast with salad

Supper   Roasted winter vegetable ratatouille (page 219) with a
baked potato *or* stir-fried vegetables with chicken and rice

Snacks   1 small bunch of grapes and 1 banana

Drink   At least 8 glasses or cups (1½ litres) of water, herbal or
fruit tea, ordinary tea or green tea. (You may also include up to
2 cups of coffee without sugar if you wish.)

Activity plan

Cardiovascular activity: Do a constant-pace workout today.
Choose your activity and aim for RPE 7, or 70 to 75 per cent MHR.

Level 1: 35 minutes

Level 2: 40 minutes

Level 3: 45 minutes

Strength/toning: This is a repeat of Day 15: perform two sets of each exercise.

Stretching: After the toning exercises, perform the stretches described on pages 150–2. Hold each stretch for 30 seconds.

Day 18

Eating plan

Breakfast   Blueberry smoothie (page 202) *or* a pot of low-fat yoghurt with fresh fruit

Lunch   Vegetable soup (page 207) with a small wholemeal pitta bread *or* a pasta and bean salad

Supper   Baked red peppers with lentils and goats' cheese (page 223) *or* a small grilled chicken breast with a baked potato, carrots and broccoli

Oaty apple crumble (page 237) *or* stewed apples

Snacks   1 orange and 1 small bowl (85g) of berries

Drink   At least 8 glasses or cups (1½ litres) of water, herbal or fruit tea, ordinary tea or green tea. (You may also include up to 2 cups of coffee without sugar if you wish.)

Activity plan

Rest day

Day 19

Eating plan

Breakfast   Fresh fruit salad with honey (page 205) *or* 1 slice of wholemeal toast with honey and fresh fruit

Lunch   Salmon and bean salad (page 212) *or* ready-bought lentil soup with a small wholemeal roll

Supper   Vegetable balti with chickpeas (page 220) and basmati rice *or* pasta and bean salad

Poached pears with cinnamon (page 238) *or* fresh pears

Snacks   2 rice cakes with peanut butter and 1 apple

Drink   At least 8 glasses or cups (1½ litres) of water, herbal or fruit tea, ordinary tea or green tea. (You may also include up to 2 cups of coffee without sugar if you wish.)

Activity plan

Rest day

Day 20

Eating plan

Breakfast   Porridge (page 203) *or* 1 small bowl whole-grain cereal with fresh fruit and skimmed milk

Lunch   Tuna and white bean salad (page 215) *or* a baked potato with tuna and sweet corn and a leafy salad

A pot of low-fat yoghurt

Supper   Grilled coconut fish (page 221) with broccoli, spinach and whole-grain rice *or* a bean and vegetable hotpot with whole-grain rice

Snacks   1 peach, a small bowl (85g) of berries, 25g (size of 4 dice) cheese

Drink   At least 8 glasses or cups (1½ litres) of water, herbal or fruit tea, ordinary tea or green tea. (You may also include up to 2 cups of coffee without sugar if you wish.)

Activity plan

Cardiovascular activity: Today you'll do another interval workout, the same as Day 15. After your warm-up do one minute at a faster pace, then one minute at a slower pace. Repeat. Aim to work at RPE 8, or 75 to 85 per cent MHR during the high-intensity intervals.

Level 1: Repeat 10 times
Level 2: Repeat 12 times
Level 3: Repeat 15 times

Strength/toning: This is a repeat of Day 15: perform two sets of each exercise.

Stretching: After the toning exercises, perform the stretches described on pages 150–2. Hold each stretch for 30 seconds.

Day 21

Eating plan

Breakfast   Tropical smoothie (page 201) *or* fresh fruit and 1 pot of low-fat yoghurt

Lunch   The perfect baked potato with a filling of your choice (page 214) *or* a large leafy salad with avocado and beans

Supper   Lentil and red pepper dahl (page 226) with whole-grain rice *or* pasta with red kidney beans and pasta sauce plus steamed broccoli

Snacks   2 satsumas, a kiwi fruit and a small handful (25g) of nuts

Drink   At least 8 glasses or cups (1½ litres) of water, herbal or fruit tea, ordinary tea or green tea. (You may also include up to 2 cups of coffee without sugar if you wish.)

Activity plan

Cardiovascular activity: It's a constant-pace workout today. Try to pick a different activity from Day 20 and aim for RPE 7, or 70 to 75 per cent MHR.

    Level 1: 35 minutes
    Level 2: 40 minutes
    Level 3: 45 minutes

Stretching: After the cardiovascular activity, perform the stretches described on pages 150–2. Hold each stretch for 30 seconds.

WEEK 4

Day 22

Eating plan

Breakfast   Fresh fruit salad with honey (page 205) *or* 1 slice of wholemeal toast with honey and fresh fruit

Lunch   Roasted herby tomato salad (page 210) *or* ready-made fresh vegetable soup with 1 slice of wholemeal bread

Supper   Pasta with chickpeas and spinach (page 224) plus carrots *or* stir-fried chicken with vegetables and whole-grain rice

Baked apples with blackberries (page 238) *or* a bowl of fresh berries

Snacks   2 satsumas; a small handful (25g) of nuts or seeds

Drink   At least 8 glasses or cups (1½ litres) of water, herbal or fruit tea, ordinary tea or green tea. (You may also include up to 2 cups of coffee without sugar if you wish.)

Activity plan

Rest day

Day 23

Eating plan

Breakfast   Cranberry orange smoothie (page 202) with 1 pot of low-fat yoghurt *or* a bowl of fresh fruit with 1 pot of yoghurt

Lunch   Chicken and lentil salad (page 213) *or* an open wholemeal sandwich topped with avocado, watercress and goats' cheese

Supper   Fish with spicy chickpeas (page 228) and a baked potato *or* vegetable and bean hotpot with whole-grain rice

Snacks   2 rice cakes with 25g (size of 4 dice) cheese; 1 pear

Drink   At least 8 glasses or cups (1½ litres) of water, herbal or fruit tea, ordinary tea or green tea. (You may also include up to 2 cups of coffee without sugar if you wish.)

Activity plan

Cardiovascular activity: Today you'll do another interval workout, this time increasing the number of intervals. After your warm-up do one minute at a faster pace, then one minute at a slower pace. Repeat. Aim to work at RPE 8, or 75 to 85 per cent MHR during the high-intensity intervals.

Level 1: Repeat 12 times
Level 2: Repeat 14 times
Level 3: Repeat 17 times

Strength/toning: This time, try to do the toning sequence 3 times, resting 20 seconds between exercises.

Stretching: After the toning exercises, perform the stretches described on pages 150–2. Hold each stretch for 30 seconds.

Day 24

Eating plan

Breakfast   Porridge (page 203) *or* 1 small bowl of bran flakes cereal with skimmed milk and a banana

Lunch   Butternut squash soup with cannellini beans (page 218) and 1 slice of wholemeal bread *or* a large leafy salad with salmon and a small wholemeal roll

Supper   Tarragon chicken breasts on lentils and mushrooms (page 229) *or* a baked potato with ratatouille and a little grated cheese with a leafy salad

Snacks   1 nectarine; 10 strawberries

Drink   At least 8 glasses or cups (1½ litres) of water, herbal or
fruit tea, ordinary tea or green tea. (You may also include up to
2 cups of coffee without sugar if you wish.)

Activity plan

Rest day

Day 25

Eating plan

Breakfast   Fruit muesli (page 204) *or* 1 slice of toast with a
poached egg and fresh fruit

Lunch   Asian prawn salad (page 212) with a small wholemeal roll
or a baked potato with baked beans and a tomato salad

Supper   Trout with roasted Mediterranean vegetables (page 222)
and a baked potato *or* a vegetable and bean curry with whole-
grain rice

Snacks   1 bowl (85g) berries, 1 apple and a small handful (25g)
of nuts or seeds

Drink   At least 8 glasses or cups (1½ litres) of water, herbal or
fruit tea, ordinary tea or green tea. (You may also include up to
2 cups of coffee without sugar if you wish.)

Activity plan

Cardiovascular activity: It's a constant-pace workout. Try to
increase your workout time another 5 minutes today. Aim for RPE 7,
or 70 to 75 per cent MHR.

Level 1: 40 minutes
Level 2: 45 minutes
Level 3: 50 minutes

Stretching: After the cardiovascular activity, perform the stretches described on pages 150–2. Hold each stretch for 30 seconds.

Day 26

Eating plan

Breakfast   A breakfast muffin (page 203) and fresh fruit *or* a small bowl of whole-grain cereal with skimmed milk and a banana

Lunch   Pitta pockets (page 215) with a leafy salad *or* ready-made fresh vegetable soup with a small wholemeal roll

Supper   Moroccan vegetable tagine (page 225) *or* a chicken and vegetable stew with potatoes
Tropical fruit salad with lime fromage frais (page 239) *or* a bowl of fresh fruit

Snacks   A small bunch of grapes and 2 apricots

Drink   At least 8 glasses or cups (1½ litres) of water, herbal or fruit tea, ordinary tea or green tea. (You may also include up to 2 cups of coffee without sugar if you wish.)

Activity plan

Rest day

Day 27

Eating plan

Breakfast   1 slice of wholemeal toast with honey and fresh
fruit *or* a blueberry smoothie (page 202) with 1 pot of low-fat
yoghurt

Lunch   Turkey and avocado sandwich (page 216) *or* a baked
potato with baked beans, a little grated cheese and a leafy
salad

Fresh fruit of your choice

Supper   Sweet-and-sour chicken with mango (page 227) with
whole-grain rice *or* grilled fish fillet with roasted Mediterranean
vegetables

Snacks   1 apple, 1 orange and a small handful (25g) of nuts

Drink   At least 8 glasses or cups (1½ litres) of water, herbal or
fruit tea, ordinary tea or green tea. (You may also include up to
2 cups of coffee without sugar if you wish.)

Activity plan

Cardiovascular activity: Today you'll do an interval workout, but
this time increasing the amount of time spent doing the intervals.
After your warm-up do two minutes at a faster pace, then two
minutes at a slower pace. Repeat. Aim to work at RPE 8, or 75 to
85 per cent MHR during the high-intensity intervals.

Level 1: Repeat 7 times

Level 2: Repeat 9 times

Level 3: Repeat 11 times

Strength/toning: Repeat the toning workout from Day 23, performing the toning sequence 3 times, resting 20 seconds between exercises.

Stretching: After the toning exercises, perform the stretches described on pages 150–2. Hold each stretch for 30 seconds.

Day 28

Eating plan

Breakfast   Porridge (page 203) *or* 1 slice of wholemeal toast with honey and fresh fruit

Lunch   Hummus with vegetable sticks (page 217) with 1 small wholemeal pitta bread *or* an open wholemeal sandwich topped with watercress, avocado and a little tuna plus a leafy salad

Supper   Roast vegetable and bean lasagne (page 230) with broccoli *or* Puy lentils with Mediterranean vegetables (page 231)

Melon and raspberries (page 240)

Snacks   2 satsumas and 2 rice cakes with peanut butter

Drink   At least 8 glasses or cups (1½ litres) of water, herbal or fruit tea, ordinary tea or green tea. (You may also include up to 2 cups of coffee without sugar if you wish.)

Activity plan

Cardiovascular activity: It's a constant-pace workout. Try to increase your workout time another 5 minutes today. Aim for RPE 7 to 8, or 75 to 85 per cent MHR.

Level 1: 45 minutes
Level 2: 50 minutes
Level 3: 55 minutes

Stretching: After the cardiovascular activity, perform the stretches described on pages 150–2. Hold each stretch for 30 seconds.

Be Slim for Life

Once you've established healthy eating and exercising habits, you need to keep them up. Carefully and gradually make the transition from eating for weight loss to eating for life.

Remember, the 28-day Plan was not a diet that you follow then stop. The idea was to show you how to integrate healthier eating habits and regular activity into your lifestyle. Following the plan will have helped establish long-term healthy habits so that eating healthily and exercising regularly become the norm from now on. So all you have to do is carry on eating the same way and making activity part of your everyday life. Because the 28-day Plan didn't ban any food group, you don't have to reintroduce certain foods or make any further changes. In fact, you've already done the hardest part by following the 28-day Plan – things will now get easier.

How to keep the weight off

Hopefully, you will have achieved many of your goals – you will have lost some weight, become fitter and feel more energetic. And you should now be feeling in better control of your eating habits. So what now?

List your achievements

Begin by writing down all your achievements. This could be the amount of weight you've lost, your new body measurements, the difference in clothes sizes, as well as subjective successes like having more energy, feeling fitter, having clearer skin, being able to run up the stairs or play with the children without feeling tired, or being able to wear fashionable clothes. Seeing how much you've accomplished will give you lots of motivation to stick to your new healthy habits.

Renew your goals

Now is a good time to revisit your goals. You may wish to revise some of them or set some new goals to help you keep the weight off. Repeat the goal-setting process you underwent before (see Chapter 1, page 26) and make a contract. Again, sign and date it and keep it somewhere prominent to keep reminding you.

Keep monitoring

If you've been keeping a food diary or a food and mood diary, don't stop! It will continue to be a useful tool helping keep you on track. It will keep you motivated and act as a warning signal if you slip back into old habits.

Evaluate

It's worthwhile evaluating what you are doing periodically. Ask yourself what's working and whether these strategies have become comfortable habits or they feel like burdens. If they have become burdensome, see if you can devise alternative strategies that will fit into your life more easily. For example, if you're struggling to maintain three one-hour gym sessions a week, you may decide to substitute some walking or cycling or exercising to a fitness DVD for some of the gym training.

Motivate

If you need to put a spark into your plan, update your motivators. You may need to renew your goals (see above) or remind yourself to reward your progress, no matter how small. Even if you have reached your weight-loss goals, you can reward yourself for reaching new fitness goals. For example, every time you complete twenty workouts, manage to swim an extra ten lengths, run an extra mile or walk an extra fifteen minutes, reward yourself. It could be with a book, a new pair of shoes, new make-up – anything that motivates you.

Be vigilant

Once you've reached your goal weight, you can begin to relax some of your restrictions, but don't relax your vigilance. Don't stop being active and don't go back to eating like a fat person. Calories still count and they always will. You should continue planning your menus, and deliberately build in the extras (you should eat a little more to maintain rather than lose weight). Act fast if you find yourself sliding back to old habits. Revive your food and activity diaries. At the first sign of things getting out of hand, stop, go back a few steps and get back in control. Reread the relevant sections of this book to remind you!

Enjoy being slim

The most important thing is to enjoy your new way of eating and exercising. Don't think of it as a permanent diet. Remember that it's what you do for most of the time that counts. It can take a while for your new healthy eating and exercising behaviour to become habits, but you will reap the benefits for a lifetime.

How to prevent lapses

You've stuck to a healthy diet with plenty of vegetables and fruit, whole grains and lean protein. And then it happens: a chocolate bar winks at you seductively from the supermarket shelf. You stumble, fall and you've blown it! But a one-time slip does not mean you are doomed to a lifetime of unhealthy eating. Missing a day or two of healthy eating is merely a short-term lapse. The important thing is to get back on track as quickly as possible. This will prevent the 'lapse' becoming a 'relapse', in which you lapse for a week or more (during which time you keep meaning to get back on track), or worse, becoming a 'collapse'. That's when you go back to old habits for a longer time and give up hope of losing weight. Here's how to nip the problem in the bud.

Distract yourself

When you get the urge to eat something unhealthy, instead of giving in straight away, wait five minutes and see if the craving goes away. During this time, distract yourself by moving to a different location – often cravings are linked to certain places or activities – going for a walk, going for a swim, or doing a different activity. If it doesn't go away, allow yourself a small amount of the food to satisfy your taste buds.

Check your hunger

Ask yourself whether you are physically hungry or emotionally hungry. If it's physical hunger you'll have a gnawing feeling in your stomach. Emotional hunger, on the other hand, tends to be for a specific food and is triggered by boredom, stress, anger or the sight and smell of appealing foods. Make sure you eat only when you are physically hungry (see page 98, on emotional hunger).

Plan ahead

Social gatherings, parties and business lunches can be high-risk situations as far as healthy eating goes. But by planning ahead, you can still enjoy these events and minimise the risk of a lapse. For example, have a small healthy snack before you go so that you won't arrive starving and be tempted to overeat. Research the menu, plan your food choices in advance – and stick to them. Once you have filled your plate, stay away from the buffet table so you won't be tempted to continue eating food you don't need. Let yourself have small portions of high-calorie treats so you don't offend anyone or feel you are missing out – but make sure it's only a small portion! If you do overindulge, balance out any excess by cutting back a little the next day and taking a bit more exercise.

What to do when you have a lapse

OK, you polished off a big hamburger and chips, and ate a whole tub of ice cream. You somehow managed to eat a day's worth of food in one sitting. And you feel like a failure. But a lapse is not a failure, so whatever you do, don't use it as an excuse to give up. Everyone has the occasional overindulgence. Forgive the slip and get back on track tomorrow.

Avoid negative self-talk

The worst thing you can do after a lapse is to think, 'I'm a slob, I'm a failure.' Such negative thoughts are driven by guilt, and will inevitably lead to further unhealthy eating – if you let them. Remember, it's what you eat and do for 80 per cent of the time that counts. You can relax the rules the remaining 20 per cent of the time and still lose weight.

Work out what went wrong

Instead of thinking of a lapse as the end of the world, think of it as a learning opportunity. Ask yourself what caused the lapse, learn from your mistakes and work out what you will do next time you find yourself in a similar situation. Was it a particular food? Don't have it in the house or, if you're in a social situation, promise yourself that you'll have only a small portion next time. Had you had a bad day and needed some comfort? Make a list of alternative activities you could do next time.

Damage limitation

If you ate too much today, you can compensate either by eating less tomorrow and/or taking a bit more exercise. Rather like managing a bank account, if you get overdrawn you need to deposit more money to bring your account back into balance. The idea is to balance your (occasional) indulgences with periods of compensation. This doesn't mean half-starving yourself, rather making an extra effort to eat more healthily and perhaps going for a thirty-minute swim/cycle/walk the next day – just enough to bring everything back into balance again.

How to survive eating out

If you are worried about eating out in case your good intentions and resolve weaken when you are confronted with an exciting menu, these tips will help steer you towards healthy choices.

1. Be the first to order so you are not swayed by other people's choices.
2. Don't skip a meal if you plan to eat out. Instead, just eat a little less. Completely skipping a meal will make you extra hungry when you arrive at the restaurant and you'll probably end up overeating.

3. Most portions served in restaurants count as two or three servings! Ask for a bag or box to take half your meal home – you won't overeat and you won't feel you've wasted your money.

4. To save calories, decide whether to have a starter or dessert but not both.

5. Steer clear of any dish described as creamy, crispy, breaded, cheesy, battered, sautéed or fried. They will be high in calories and fat. Instead look for boiled, grilled, poached, stir-fried or baked.

6. Start with a salad – it's a low-calorie-dense meal so it'll fill you up and take the edge off your appetite. Choose a low-calorie dressing and ask for dressing on the side.

7. Avoid the bread basket – bread has a medium calorie density but is too easy to over-consume when you are ravenous.

8. Alternatively, start with a clear or vegetable soup (avoid anything creamy), as the fibre and water fill you up for relatively few calories.

9. Request a starter or child's portion of a main dish.

10. Ask the waiter to substitute salad or vegetables for high-fat items such as chips or fries.

11. Choose main dishes that include plenty of vegetables or order extra vegetable side dishes (plain, not fried or smothered in butter or cream) to complement your main dish.

12. Order fresh fruit or sorbet for dessert. If you can't resist a richer dessert, share it with a friend.

13. Share a main course with a friend and order your own salads or extra side dishes of vegetables to fill you up. It's more economical and better for you.

14. Save calories by limiting the amount of alcohol you have (and too much alcohol weakens your resolve to make healthy choices).

15. Slow your eating by trying to keep pace with the slowest eater at the table. Take time to savour the flavours of the meal and enjoy the company you are with.

Eating out guide to restaurants

Chinese menus

1. Many of the menu options are not only high in fat but are also laden with sugar and salt.
2. Avoid anything with the words 'battered', 'deep fried' or 'crispy'. Instead, order steamed dishes, chop suey, stir-fried vegetables and boiled instead of fried rice.
3. Avoid sweet-and-sour pork with egg-fried rice (the most popular choice in UK), which provides a staggering 60g of fat and 1,330 calories.
4. Avoid crispy duck with its 650 calories and 36g fat per 4 pancakes.
5. Lychees are a good low-fat choice for dessert.

Beware of	Better bets
Crispy duck	Soup
Sweet-and-sour pork	Vegetable, chicken or prawn
Spare ribs	chop suey
Prawn crackers	Sweet-and-sour vegetables
Fried noodles	Stir-fried vegetables
Egg-fried rice	Boiled rice and noodles
	Szechwan prawns

Indian menus

1. Steer clear of kormas, pasandas and masalas, which usually contain oil, cream or ghee (clarified butter).
2. Dry-cooked dishes such as tandooris and tikka are likely to be lower in fat.
3. Bhunas, dopiaza, vindaloos and madras dishes are likely to be lower in fat than those in richer sauces.
4. Avoid rogan josh, biryanis and jaipuris, as they are high in fat.
5. Vegetable balti, dahl (lentils) or aloo gobi (potato and cauliflower curry) with boiled rice make good vegetarian options.
6. Go for chapattis made without fat, which contain 11g less fat and 130 fewer calories per portion than chapattis with fat.
7. Go halves on naan bread – a whole one packs 20g fat and 540 calories.
8. Avoid chicken tikka masala (the most popular dish on the menu in the UK) – it typically provides 860 calories and 47g fat.

Beware of	Better bets
Samosas	Chapatti, plain naan
Anything fried	Chicken tikka
Most meat curries and biryanis	Tandoori dishes
Chicken tikka masala	Chickpea dishes (e.g. channa
Anything in a korma, pasanda or	dahl)
masala sauce	Lentil dishes (e.g. dahl)
Rogan josh	Dry vegetable curries
Lamb pasanda	Vegetable side dishes
	Aloo gobi

Pizza and pasta menus

1. Ignore the meal deals that tempt you to eat gigantic portions plus extra garlic bread and gallons of fizzy drink.
2. Share a pizza – a whole one typically provides 1,000 to 1,400 calories and up to 60g of fat.
3. Opt for pizza with extra vegetable toppings and goat's cheese rather than mozzarella.
4. Avoid meat toppings like pepperoni, ham, sausage, ground beef and pork – they are loaded with fat and salt.
5. Avoid pizzas with a stuffed crust and toppings that go right to the edge – they can add an extra 200 calories and 15g of fat to your pizza.
6. Choose minestrone soup or a tomato salad for starters instead of garlic bread.
7. Choose simple tomato or vegetable sauces for pasta.
8. Avoid high-fat cream, carbonara or cheese sauces.

Beware of	Better bets
Pasta with creamy/buttery sauces	Pasta with tomato-, vegetable- or seafood-based sauces
Pasta with Bolognese sauce	Pasta filled with spinach/ricotta
Lasagne (meat)	Gnocchi with tomato-based sauce
Pizza with meat, pepperoni, salami or extra cheese toppings	Pizza with vegetable toppings
Garlic bread, dough sticks	Salads: tomatoes, avocado, olives
Tiramisu	Vegetable risottos
	Crème caramel and gelati

Burger Restaurants

1. Go for the smallest portion available: the bigger the burger and fries the more calories and fat you get.
2. A plain hamburger supplies around 253 calories and 7.7g fat but a larger version contains between 500 and 800 calories plus 23–50g fat.
3. Go for a chicken salad without dressing – it contains around 300 calories and 11g fat.
4. Omit mayonnaise, sauces and dressings (or ask for small portions).

Beware of	Better bets
Large/quarterpounder hamburgers	Plain grilled hamburger
Chicken burgers	Flame-grilled chicken
Chicken nuggets	Salad, e.g. chicken Caesar salad
Chips/fries	Fruit
Anything fried	Grilled chicken sandwich
Doughnuts	
Apple pies	

Greek menus

1. Low-fat dips such as tzatziki and hummus are good options.
2. Fill up with salads such as Greek salad, tomatoes or taboulleh.
3. Stuffed vine leaves, couscous and lentil dishes are healthy.
4. Avoid rich meat-based dishes.
5. Opt for kebabs served with salad or grilled fish dishes.

Beware of	Better bets
Moussaka	Greek salad
Taramasalata	Tomato or cucumber salad
Lamb dishes	Tzatziki and pitta bread
Keftethakia (meat balls)	Hummus
Baklava	Grilled fish
	Dolmades
	Stuffed tomatoes
	Fresh fruit

Mexican menus

1. Many items on the menu are deep fried so can be very high in calories and fat.
2. For starters opt for guacamole and raw vegetable crudités; avoid potato skins and fried tortilla chips.
3. Order chicken or vegetable fajitas (soft flour tortillas).
4. Steer clear of enchiladas or burritos (which are fried and therefore loaded with fat).
5. Avoid the sour cream that accompanies many main dishes.
6. Avoid tortillas as they are often softened in oil and deep fried.
7. Choose small portions of refried beans – they can be mixed with fat and cheese and are also very salty.
8. Try grilled fish or chicken with a salad.

Beware of	Better bets
Tortilla chips	Guacamole
Potato skins	Bean burritos and tortillas
Beef chilli	Vegetable or chicken fajitas
Tortillas/burritos with meat	Tostadas with beans or
Chimichangas	vegetables
Chicken, beef or vegetable	Vegetable chilli
enchiladas	

Japanese menus

1. Sushi, teriyaki sahimi and sukiyaki are all good low-fat choices.
2. Opt for clear miso soup with vegetables or noodles.
3. Soba noodles, made from buckwheat, are a healthy option.
4. Steer clear of anything described as tempura, which means deep fried.
5. Choose boiled rather than fried rice.

Beware of	Better bets
Fried rice	Miso soup
Tempura dishes	Seaweed dishes
	Soba noodles
	Nori rolls
	Chicken or beef teriyaki
	Sushi
	Sashimi
	Sukiyaki

Help – I'm stuck on a plateau

If you find yourself on a weight-loss plateau, it could be that you've been fooling yourself that you're eating less than you really are. It's easy to subconsciously overeat – sampling food while you're cooking, clearing up the leftovers, eating snacks on the move, or eating while watching TV.

Monitor your food intake

Keep a daily food diary and start writing down everything you've eaten, not forgetting the odd biscuit, the glass of wine after work, the handful of crisps while watching a film with your family, the forkful of cheesecake from your friend's slice. You'll soon find the explanation for your weight-loss plateau. If you find it too hard to do all the time, try monitoring your intake only at problem times, say at weekends or when travelling.

Renew your support

This is a time when you need to call on the support of your family and friends, the ones you identified at the start of your journey (see Chapter 1, page 32). They can encourage you to stick with your healthy eating and activity plans when you find it hard to keep going.

Revisit your goals

Plateaus often happen when you lose sight of your goals. Perhaps you've stopped reading your goals, in which case, place them somewhere prominent where you'll see them every day as a constant reminder. Perhaps you've set yourself an unrealistic goal and are frustrated about your lack of progress. Revise your goal or break the goal into smaller short-term goals.

Eating to stay slim – a summary

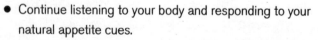

- Continue listening to your body and responding to your natural appetite cues.
- Opt mainly for foods with a low calorie density and limit portion sizes of those foods with a high calorie density.
- Include as many foods as possible with a high satiety rating.
- Continue taking responsibility for your eating habits, being honest with yourself and learning from past mistakes.
- Remember to believe in yourself and develop your self-esteem.
- Work on developing a positive mindset when it comes to food and activity – changing your old beliefs doesn't happen overnight, it can take months of practice.
- Follow the 80/20 rule: it's what you do MOST of the time – i.e. 80 per cent – that counts.
- Don't deny forbidden foods – allow yourself to eat what you want but decide beforehand how much you are going to have.

- Never feel guilty about food. Even if you overeat one day just get back on track the next day. Eat a little less at your next meal or the next day or take a bit more exercise.
- Reward yourself when you have reached a goal.
- Monitor your progress and write down what you're eating and what you're doing – keeping a daily food and activity diary will help keep your motivation level high.
- Be organised so you will always have healthy food around. Plan your menus a few days in advance and make shopping lists – preparing and eating healthy food will feel less of an effort.
- When eating out, eat satisfying portions of vegetable dishes such as soup, vegetable curries, salads and stir-fries. If necessary, order extra vegetables or salad to reduce the calorie density of your meal.
- Remember always to enjoy your food.

Exercising to stay slim – a summary

- Repeat part or all of the activity plan. If you wish to get faster results, you should gradually increase either the amount of time you exercise, the frequency or the intensity. For example, if you were at level 1, progress to level 2; if you were at level 2, progress to level 3.
- To challenge yourself further, you could perform more interval cardiovascular workouts in place of steady-pace workouts.
- Keep your motivation levels high by varying your workouts.

Change the type of cardiovascular exercise you do – try new activities or sports.

- Ask a personal trainer to devise an exercise programme suited to your individual goals, either on an occasional or regular basis. To find a trainer, ask a friend for a recommendation or find one in your area from the National Register of Personal Trainers (www.nrpt.co.uk). You can also check the qualifications of your exercise teacher on the Register of Exercise Professionals (www.exerciseregister.org).

- Keeping an activity diary will help you track your progress and keep you motivated.

- Remember, activity isn't just for fat-burning, so don't give up once you have reached your weight-loss goal. It keeps your heart healthy, strengthens and tones your body, and helps reduce stress.

- Include all three types of activity: cardiovascular activity, strength/toning exercises and stretching. Each provides different benefits and all three are important for overall fitness and good health.

The Recipes

Breakfast recipes

Strawberry banana smoothie

Makes 2 drinks

> 250ml (8fl.oz) orange juice
> 125g (4oz) strawberries
> 2 bananas, frozen and sliced

1. Place the orange juice, strawberries and frozen banana slices in a smoothie maker, blender or food processor and process until smooth and thick.
2. Serve immediately.

Tropical smoothie

Makes 2 drinks

> About 10 ice cubes
> Juice and zest of 1 lime
> 125g (4oz) strawberries
> 125g (4oz) fresh pineapple
> ½ a mango, peeled and roughly chopped
> ¼ of a Galia melon, peeled and chopped
> 1 banana, peeled and roughly chopped

1. Place the ice cubes in the goblet of a smoothie maker, blender or food processor and process until slushy.
2. Add the remaining ingredients, in batches if necessary, and blend until smooth.
3. Serve in chilled glasses immediately.

Blueberry smoothie

Makes 2 drinks

125g (4oz) raspberries
125g (4oz) blueberries
1 small banana, peeled and cut into chunks
125ml (4fl.oz) fresh orange juice
A cupful of crushed ice

1. Place the ingredients in a smoothie maker, blender or food processor and blend until smooth and frothy.
2. Serve immediately.

Cranberry orange smoothie

Makes 2 drinks

A small cupful of crushed ice
250ml (8fl.oz) cranberry juice drink
60g (2oz) raspberries
150ml (5fl.oz) orange juice

1. Place the ingredients in a smoothie maker, blender or food processor and blend until smooth and frothy.
2. Serve immediately.

Porridge

Makes 1 serving

> 60g (2oz) porridge oats
>
> 350ml (12fl.oz) skimmed milk
>
> Chopped fresh fruit, such as sliced banana, blueberries or strawberries
>
> 25g (1oz) dried fruit e.g. raisins, dates or figs
>
> 2tsp honey

1. Mix the oats and milk. Cook in a microwave for about 4 minutes, stirring halfway through, or in a saucepan for about 5 minutes, stirring continuously.
2. Top with the fresh and dried fruit. Drizzle with honey.

Breakfast muffins

Makes 12 muffins

> 125g (4oz) white self-raising flour
>
> 125g (4oz) wholemeal self-raising flour
>
> 1tbsp (15ml) oil
>
> 40g (1½oz) soft brown sugar
>
> 1 egg
>
> 150ml (5fl.oz) skimmed milk
>
> 60g (2oz) chopped dates or raisins

1. Preheat the oven to 220°C/425°F/Gas mark 7.
2. Mix the flours together in a bowl. Add the oil, sugar, egg and milk. Mix well.
3. Stir in the dried fruit.

4. Spoon into a nonstick muffin tray and bake for about 15 minutes until golden brown.

Fruit muesli

Makes 4 servings

175g (6oz) oats
300ml (½ pint) skimmed milk
2tbsp sultanas
2tbsp toasted flaked almonds, chopped hazelnuts or cashews
225g (8oz) fruit, e.g. bananas, blueberries, strawberries, raspberries
1 apple, peeled and grated
1tbsp honey

1. In a large bowl, mix together the oats, milk, sultanas and nuts. Cover and leave overnight in the fridge.
2. Just before serving, stir in the fruit, grated apple and honey. Spoon into cereal bowls.

Yoghurt with dried fruit compote

Makes 4 servings

Zest and juice of 1 orange
2tbsp (30ml) acacia honey
300ml (½ pint) water
150ml (5fl.oz) orange juice
85g (3oz) dried figs, halved
85g (3oz) dried apricots

85g (3oz) pitted prunes

450ml pot natural bio-yoghurt or fat-free Greek-style yoghurt

1. Combine the zest, freshly squeezed juice, honey, water and orange juice in a saucepan. Bring the mixture to the boil, stirring until the honey is dissolved, then add the dried fruit and simmer, covered, for about 15 minutes until they become plump and soft. Allow to cool and keep covered in the fridge until you are ready to serve.
2. Divide the yoghurt between 4 bowls. Top with the fruit compote.

Fresh fruit salad with honey

Makes 2 servings

4tbsp (60ml) hot water

1tbsp (15ml) acacia (or clear) honey

175g (6oz) berry fruits, e.g. strawberries, raspberries, blueberries

1 banana, peeled and sliced

2 kiwi fruit, peeled, cut into ½-inch pieces

125g (4oz) seedless grapes

1. Dissolve the honey in the hot water in a large bowl.
2. Prepare the berry fruit, slicing into bite-sized pieces, if necessary.
3. Add all the fruit to the honey syrup in the bowl. Toss to combine. Cover and chill until you are ready to serve.

Lunch Recipes

Spicy couscous salad

Makes 4 servings

- 250g (9oz) couscous
- 400ml (13fl.oz) hot vegetable stock or water
- ½ a red pepper
- ½ a yellow pepper
- 1 red onion, sliced
- 10–12 cherry tomatoes, halved
- 2tbsp (30ml) extra-virgin olive oil
- ½tsp cumin seeds
- A small handful of fresh coriander, chopped
- 1tbsp lemon juice
- A little low-sodium salt and freshly ground black pepper

1. Put the couscous in a large bowl and cover with the hot stock or water. Stir briefly, cover and allow to stand for 5 minutes until the stock has been absorbed. Fluff up with a fork.
2. Remove the seeds from the peppers and cut them into wide strips. Place in a large roasting tin with the onion slices and cherry tomatoes, drizzle over the olive oil, scatter over the cumin seeds and toss lightly so that the vegetables are well coated in the oil. Roast in the oven for about 15 minutes until the peppers are slightly charred on the outside and tender in the middle. Allow to cool, then roughly chop the peppers.
3. Add the roasted vegetables (with the cumin seeds), coriander and lemon juice to the couscous. Season to taste with the low-sodium salt and black pepper. Stir well to combine and serve.

Moroccan-style lentil soup

Makes 4 servings

  2tbsp olive oil
  1 onion, sliced
  2 leeks, sliced
  2 carrots, sliced
  2 stalks celery, thinly sliced
  2 potatoes, diced
  1½ litres vegetable stock
  175g (6oz) red lentils
  2tsp harissa paste
  Juice of ½ a lemon
  2tbsp chopped fresh flat-leaf parsley

1. Heat the olive oil in a large heavy-based saucepan. Add the onion, leeks, carrots, celery and potato and cook gently for about 10 minutes or until the vegetables have softened, but not coloured.
2. Add the lentils and harissa. Pour in the stock and bring to the boil. Simmer, partially covered, for a further 15 to 20 minutes until the vegetables and lentils are tender.
3. Add the lemon juice, season to taste with a little salt and black pepper and stir in the fresh parsley.

Vegetable soup

Makes 4 servings

  1tbsp (15ml) extra-virgin olive oil

1 onion, finely sliced

450g (1lb) carrots, sliced

225g (8oz) parsnips, diced

1 litre (1¾ pints) vegetable stock

1 bay leaf

125g (4oz) green beans, topped, tailed and halved

125g (4oz) frozen peas

A small handful of basil leaves, roughly torn

A little low-sodium salt and freshly ground black pepper

1. Heat the olive oil in a heavy-based saucepan over a moderate heat. Add the onion and cook gently for about 5 minutes until softened.

2. Add the carrots and parsnips to the pan and continue to cook over a moderate heat for 5 minutes, stirring occasionally, until the vegetables soften a little.

3. Add the stock and bay leaf and bring to the boil. Simmer for 10 minutes, add the beans and peas and cook for a further 5 minutes.

4. Remove and discard the bay leaf. Liquidise the soup using a hand blender or conventional blender. Stir in the basil and season with low-sodium salt and freshly ground pepper.

Rocket and courgette frittata with warm tomato sauce

Makes 4 servings

4 medium courgettes, sliced (about 500g)

3tbsp olive oil

8 eggs
1 tbsp fresh thyme, chopped
A handful of rocket
300g (10oz) vine cherry tomatoes, halved
1 clove garlic, crushed
Extra rocket to serve

1. Preheat the oven to 230°C/450°F/Gas mark 8.
2. Place the courgette slices in a large roasting tin and toss with 1 tbsp of the olive oil. Roast for 12 to 15 minutes or until tender. Remove from the oven and preheat the grill to high.
3. Meanwhile, beat the eggs in a bowl with the thyme. Stir the courgettes and rocket into the egg mixture.
4. Heat 1 tbsp of olive oil in a 25cm nonstick frying pan and add the egg mixture. Cook until puffed up around the edges, then turn the heat to low and cook for 10 to 12 minutes until the frittata has set around the edges but not on top.
5. Place under the preheated grill and cook for 3 to 4 minutes until the top is set. Remove from the grill and transfer to a large flat plate.
6. Meanwhile, place the cherry tomatoes, garlic, and the remaining 1 tbsp olive oil in a small saucepan and season. Place over a medium heat and warm through gently for 5 minutes until the tomatoes have softened and released their juice. Serve a wedge of the frittata with a spoonful of warm tomato sauce and extra rocket.

Roasted herby tomato salad

Makes 4 servings

8 large English vine tomatoes, halved
1 tbsp fresh thyme, leaves removed
2 cloves garlic, crushed
1 tbsp extra-virgin olive oil
Freshly ground black pepper
60g (2oz) wholemeal breadcrumbs
1 tbsp fresh flat-leaf parsley, finely chopped
100g (3½oz) bag of rocket
A little balsamic vinegar

1. Preheat the oven to 180°C/360°F/Gas mark 4. Place the tomatoes on a baking tray, cut-side up. Scatter over the thyme leaves and half the garlic, drizzle with the olive oil and season with a little black pepper. Roast for 15 minutes or until softened, then remove from the oven.

2. Meanwhile, cook the breadcrumbs in a nonstick frying pan over a gentle heat with the remaining garlic for 2 to 3 minutes, stirring occasionally, until the crumbs are golden. Remove from the heat and leave to cool. Stir in the parsley.

3. Place a mound of rocket in the centres of 4 serving plates. Arrange 4 roast tomato halves on each plate.

4. Drizzle a little balsamic vinegar around the tomatoes and then scatter the breadcrumb topping over. Serve warm or cold.

Asparagus and broad bean salad with poached egg

Makes 4 servings

225g (8oz) asparagus spears
150g (5oz) broad beans
150g (5oz) watercress
2tbsp olive oil
1tbsp pumpkinseed oil
1tbsp lemon juice
4 eggs
60g (2oz) toasted pumpkinseeds

1. Trim the asparagus spears. Cook for 2 minutes then add the broad beans and simmer for a further 3 minutes until both are just tender. Drain and allow them to cool.
2. To make the dressing, shake the olive oil, pumpkinseed oil and the lemon juice in a bottle or screw-top glass jar.
3. Mix the cooled vegetables and washed watercress with the dressing. Divide between 4 bowls.
4. To poach the eggs, bring a large pan of water to boil. Break an egg into a teacup then gently slip the egg into the water. Do the same with the other eggs then simmer very gently for 1 minute. Turn off the heat, cover and leave to sit for 5 minutes until the eggs are just set.
5. Lift the eggs from the water using a slotted spoon, drain well, and then place 1 on top of each salad. Scatter over the pumpkinseeds and serve immediately.

Salmon and bean salad

Makes 4 servings

150g (5oz) salad leaves

420g (14oz) can mixed beans, drained and rinsed

4tbsp low-fat vinaigrette dressing

2tbsp fresh chopped parsley

Freshly ground black pepper

213g (7oz) can wild red salmon, drained

200g (7oz) cherry tomatoes, halved

4 spring onions, chopped

1. Arrange the salad leaves on 4 plates. Mix the beans with the vinaigrette, parsley and freshly ground black pepper.
2. Remove the skin and bones from the salmon and lightly flake the flesh. Mix with the tomatoes, spring onions and the bean mixture. Heap on top of the salad leaves.

Asian prawn salad

Makes 4 servings

125g (4oz) mangetout

4 spring onions

150g (5oz) cucumber

225g (8oz) cooked tiger prawns

125g bag of salad leaves

2.5cm (1-inch) piece of root ginger, peeled and grated

1 clove garlic, crushed

1 small red chilli, seeded and finely chopped

1tbsp caster sugar
Juice of 1 lime
2tbsp rice vinegar
1tbsp sunflower oil

1. Cook the mangetout in boiling water for 1 minute. Drain, rinse in cold water then drain again. Slice the mangetout and place in a bowl. Slice the spring onions and cucumber and combine with the mangetout.
2. Add the prawns and salad leaves and toss together.
3. Place the ginger, garlic, chilli, sugar, lime juice, vinegar and oil in a bottle or screw-top jar and shake together. Pour over the salad and toss gently.

Chicken and lentil salad

Makes 4 servings

2tbsp olive oil
4 chicken breast fillets, sliced
1 clove garlic, crushed
1 small onion, chopped
410g (14oz) can lentils, drained and rinsed
3 or 4 tomatoes, finely chopped
2tbsp lemon juice
1tbsp clear honey
2tbsp fresh flat-leaf parsley, roughly chopped

1. Heat 1tbsp of the olive oil in a large frying pan over a high heat and sauté the chicken for 5 or 6 minutes or until cooked and

there is no pink meat. Add the garlic, onion, lentils and tomatoes and cook, stirring, for about 2 minutes until heated.

2. For the dressing, shake together the remaining olive oil, lemon juice and honey in a bottle or screw-top jar. Stir the dressing and half the parsley into the lentils in the pan. Transfer to a serving dish, scatter over the remaining parsley and serve warm.

The perfect baked potato

Makes 4 servings

> 4 large (225–275g) potatoes – Maris Piper, King Edward, Desiree or Cara are especially good varieties for baking

1. Preheat the oven to 220°C/425°F/Gas mark 7.
2. Scrub and prick the potatoes in several places with a fork.
3. For crisp skins, leave as they are, or roll, while still damp, in coarse sea salt. Alternatively, wrap the potatoes in foil – this keeps them moist and will soften the skins.
4. Put the potatoes on a baking sheet. Bake for 1–1½ hours according to size. Test by squeezing; the potato will feel soft when cooked.
5. With a sharp knife, make a deep cross on top and press firmly in a cloth until all four points open out. Top with your chosen filling (see below).
6. Alternatively, cut the potatoes in half lengthways, scoop out the soft potato into a bowl (put the skins back into the oven to crisp up) and mash with seasoning, then add the filling of your choice and spoon back into the skins for serving.

Choose any of the following fillings: baked beans, cheddar cheese, mozzarella cheese, plain yoghurt, salsa, stir-fried vegetables, chicken mixed with a little mayonnaise, hummus, cottage cheese, prawns, ratatouille, dahl (see page 226), tuna mixed with plain yoghurt or mayonnaise, grilled mushrooms, scrambled egg and tomato, sweet corn.

Tuna and white bean salad

Makes 4 servings

125g (4oz) ready-washed watercress
400g (14oz) tinned haricot or cannellini beans, drained and rinsed
200g (7oz) tin of tuna in spring water, drained
2 celery stalks, finely chopped
Handful of flat-leaf parsley, chopped
2tbsp (30ml) extra virgin olive oil
1tbsp (15ml) lemon juice
1 clove of garlic, finely chopped
Lemon wedges to serve

1. Place the watercress on a large serving plate. In a separate bowl, combine the beans and the tuna, roughly breaking the tuna up into large flakes. Add the celery and parsley.
2. Shake the olive oil, lemon juice and garlic in a bottle or screw-top glass jar, then drizzle over the bean mixture. Toss well and pile on top of the watercress. Serve with lemon wedges.

Pitta pockets

Makes 4 pockets

2 skinless chicken breast fillets
1tbsp olive oil

A little low-sodium salt and freshly ground black pepper

Lemon wedges

4 wholemeal pitta breads

1 pack mixed-leaf salad

1. Brush the chicken breasts with olive oil and season with low-sodium salt and pepper. Place on a hot griddle pan, or under a grill, and cook for 5 to 8 minutes on each side, or until thoroughly cooked.

2. Meanwhile, warm the pitta breads under the grill or in the oven. When the chicken is cooked, cut into thin slices.

3. Cut the pitta breads along one side and open out to form pockets. Divide the mixed-leaf salad between the four pittas and top with the grilled chicken. Garnish with the lemon wedges.

Turkey and avocado sandwich

Makes 4 servings

8 slices wholemeal bread

1 clove garlic, halved

25g (1oz) olive oil spread

1 large, ripe avocado

Juice of ½ a lime

150g (5oz) cooked turkey, thinly sliced

1tbsp chopped fresh coriander

1 large tomato, sliced

100g (3½oz) pack of lamb's lettuce (or other salad leaves)

1. Rub the bread with the halved garlic clove, and then spread the bread with the olive oil spread. Peel the avocado and remove the

stone. Roughly mash half the avocado with the lime juice and
thinly slice the other half.

2. Spread the mashed avocado over two slices of bread, then
   season. Layer the sliced avocado and turkey on top, and then
   scatter over the coriander.
3. Finish with slices of tomato and lamb's lettuce. Top with the
   remaining bread and press down gently. Secure with cocktail
   sticks. Cut in half and serve.

Hummus with vegetable sticks

Makes 4 servings

400g (14oz) tinned chickpeas
1 or 2 garlic cloves, crushed
2tbsp (30ml) extra-virgin olive oil
1tbsp (15ml) tahini (sesame seed paste)
Juice of ½ a lemon
2–4 tbsp (30–60ml) water
A little low-sodium salt and freshly ground black pepper
For the vegetable sticks:
Carrots, celery, cucumber, peppers cut into batons
Baby sweet corn
Cherry tomatoes

1. Drain and rinse the chickpeas. Put the remainder in a food
   processor or blender with the garlic, olive oil, tahini, lemon juice
   and water. Whiz until smooth, add a little low-sodium salt and
   freshly ground black pepper and process again. Taste to check

the seasoning. Add extra water if necessary to give the desired consistency.

2. Spoon into a shallow dish and drizzle over a few drops of olive oil. Chill in the fridge for at least 2 hours before serving. Serve with vegetable sticks of your choice.

Butternut squash soup with cannellini beans

Makes 4 servings

1 small onion
½ a medium butternut squash
2 carrots, sliced
1 garlic clove, crushed
1tsp (5ml) grated fresh ginger
Pinch of freshly grated nutmeg (optional)
500ml (16fl.oz) vegetable stock
1tbsp (15ml) olive oil
410g (14oz) can cannellini beans, drained and rinsed
A little low-sodium salt and freshly ground black pepper

1. Peel and chop the onion. Peel the butternut squash and cut the flesh into chunks.
2. Place the vegetables, garlic, and grated ginger, optional nutmeg and vegetable stock in a large saucepan. Bring to the boil, lower the heat, cover and simmer for about 20 minutes until the vegetables are tender.
3. Remove from the heat and liquidise with the oil until smooth using a blender, food processor or hand blender.
4. Return to the saucepan, add the cannellini beans and heat

through again. Season the soup with the low-sodium salt and freshly ground black pepper.

Supper Recipes

Roasted winter vegetable ratatouille

Makes 4 servings

 2 onions, cut into thick slices
 1 red pepper, deseeded and sliced
 ½ a butternut squash, peeled and cubed
 2 parsnips, peeled and cut into chunks
 2 cloves of garlic, crushed
 2×400g (14oz) cans cherry tomatoes
 2tbsp (30ml) extra-virgin olive oil
 A little low-sodium salt and freshly ground black pepper
 2tbsp (30ml) basil leaves or chopped fresh parsley
 Drizzle of balsamic vinegar

1. Preheat the oven to 200°C/400°F/Gas mark 6. Place the prepared vegetables and garlic in a large roasting tin. Drizzle over the olive oil and toss lightly so that the vegetables are well coated in the oil.

2. Roast in the oven for about 30 minutes until the vegetables are slightly charred on the outside and tender in the middle. Remove from the oven, add the cherry tomatoes and 500ml water. Cover the tin with foil and cook for a further 60 minutes, stirring occasionally until the vegetables are tender. Season to taste with low-sodium salt and freshly ground black pepper and stir in the

fresh herbs and balsamic vinegar. Serve hot or cold with baked potatoes or brown rice.

Vegetable balti with chickpeas

Makes 4 servings

    2tbsp (30ml) olive oil
    1 onion, sliced
    2 carrots, sliced
    ½ a cauliflower, broken into small florets
    125g (4oz) broccoli florets
    60g (2oz) green beans
    1×400g jar tikka masala cooking sauce
    300ml (½ pint) water
    200g (7oz) basmati rice
    100g (3½oz) ready-washed spinach
    225g (8oz) tinned chickpeas, rinsed and drained
    Small handful of fresh coriander leaves, chopped

1. Heat the oil in a large pan and add the onion. Cook gently for 5 minutes until softened. Add the carrots, cauliflower, broccoli and beans, and cook for a further 2 to 3 minutes before adding the sauce and water. Bring to the boil, cover and simmer for 15 to 20 minutes, stirring occasionally, until the vegetables are tender.
2. Meanwhile, cook the rice according to the packet instructions. Drain and add to the curry with the spinach and chickpeas. Cook for a further 2 to 3 minutes.
3. Stir in the coriander. Serve topped with a little natural yoghurt.

Grilled coconut fish

Makes 4 servings

4 fillets of firm white fish e.g. halibut, haddock, monkfish or
 Icelandic cod
2tsp green curry paste
1tsp grated fresh ginger
3tbsp chopped fresh parsley
3tbsp coconut cream

1. Preheat the grill to a high temperature. Place the fish fillets on a
    lightly oiled baking tray. Grill for about 4 minutes.
2. Meanwhile, make a paste by combining the green curry paste,
    ginger, parsley and coconut cream.
3. Turn the fish fillets over and brush the paste over each. Return to
    the grill and cook for about 5 to 7 minutes or until the paste is
    slightly coloured.
4. Serve with lemon or lime wedges.

Chicken roasted with butternut squash

Makes 4 servings

1 butternut squash
A little extra-virgin olive oil
4 chicken breasts on the bone
A little low-sodium salt and freshly ground black pepper
2tbsp chopped fresh thyme (or 2tsp dried thyme)

1. Heat the oven to 200°C/400°F/Gas mark 6.
2. Peel the butternut squash and cut the flesh into 5mm slices.

Cover the base of a baking tin with the squash slices, drizzle over a little oil, then scatter with thyme and season with black pepper.

3. Place the chicken breasts over the squash, drizzle over a little olive oil, then turn so they are well coated with oil.

4. Cook the chicken and the squash in the oven for 20 to 30 minutes, depending on the size of the chicken breasts, until the chicken is golden. The squash should be soft but not mushy.

5. Serve with steamed green beans.

Trout with roasted Mediterranean vegetables

Makes 4 servings

2 small bulbs of fennel

2 red peppers

2 courgettes

1 red onion

200g (7oz) cherry tomatoes

About 12 black olives

3tbsp (45ml) extra-virgin olive oil

2 garlic cloves, crushed

A few sprigs of rosemary

2 lemons, cut into 8 wedges

4 medium trout, about 350g (12oz) each

250ml (8fl.oz) white wine

1. Preheat the oven to 200°C/400°F/Gas mark 6.

2. Cut the fennel bulbs into halves or quarters, depending on size. Remove the seeds from the peppers and cut them into wide strips. Cut the red onion into wedges. Slice the courgette.

3. Place the prepared vegetables, tomatoes and olives in a large roasting tin with the garlic, rosemary and lemon wedges. Drizzle over the olive oil and toss lightly so that the vegetables are well coated in the oil. Place the trout on top of the vegetables.

4. Pour the wine over the trout and vegetables and season with low-sodium salt and black pepper. Cover the dish with foil and roast in the oven for about 30 minutes until the vegetables are slightly charred on the outside and tender in the middle.

Baked red peppers with lentils and goats' cheese

Makes 4 servings

4 medium red peppers
2tbsp olive oil
250g (9oz) pack ready-cooked puy lentils (or tinned)
85g (3oz) baby plum tomatoes, halved
100g (3½oz) goats' cheese, sliced
2tbsp fresh basil leaves, roughly torn

1. Heat the oven to 190°C/375°F/Gas mark 5.
2. Cut the peppers in half lengthways, keeping the stalk attached, and remove the seeds. Brush the outsides with a little of the olive oil then place them, skin-side down, in a roasting tin, packed quite tightly so they don't roll over.
3. Spoon the lentils into the pepper halves and top with the tomatoes and goats' cheese pieces. Drizzle over the remaining olive oil and season. Bake in the oven for 20 to 25 minutes, or until the peppers are soft.

4. Scatter over the basil leaves and serve immediately with a leafy salad and new potatoes.

Pasta with chickpeas and spinach

Makes 4 servings

410g can chickpeas, drained and rinsed
350g (12oz) tub fresh tomato pasta sauce
400g (14oz) fresh penne pasta
200g (7oz) bag fresh spinach
Freshly ground black pepper
25g (1oz) parmesan shavings
Olive oil, to drizzle

1. Place the chickpeas in a medium pan with the tomato sauce and 100ml cold water. Bring to the boil over a low heat. Turn off the heat and cover.
2. Meanwhile, bring a large pan of water to the boil. Add the pasta and return to the boil for 5 minutes or until the pasta is just tender. Drain thoroughly. Stir in the spinach and allow to wilt.
3. Place the pasta in a serving dish and pour the hot pasta sauce and chickpea mixture over the top, then toss together and season with black pepper. Top each serving with Parmesan shavings and a drizzle of olive oil.

Vegetable stir-fry with sesame noodles

Makes 4 servings

1tsp clear honey
Juice of 1 large orange

3tbsp dark soy sauce

2tbsp sunflower oil

1 onion, sliced

1 large carrot, peeled and cut into thin strips

225g (8oz) pak-choi or spring cabbage, shredded

2.5cm piece root ginger, peeled and grated

1 clove garlic, crushed

225g (8oz) ready-cooked egg noodles

3tbsp sesame seeds, toasted

1. In a small bowl, mix together the honey, orange juice and soy sauce and set aside.

2. Heat the oil in a wok or large frying pan. Add the onion and carrot and stir-fry for 2 to 3 minutes. Add the pak-choi or cabbage, ginger and garlic and stir-fry for a further 2 to 3 minutes.

3. Add the ready-cooked egg noodles to the wok and pour in the spicy-sauce mix. Toss everything together and cook for a further 2 to 3 minutes, or until piping hot. Scatter with the toasted sesame seeds and serve at once.

Moroccan vegetable tagine

Makes 4 servings

2tbsp olive oil

1 onion, sliced

1 large aubergine, cut into 3cm cubes

½tsp ground cumin

½tsp ground coriander

½tsp ground cinnamon

1 lemon
2 large courgettes, cut into thin batons
2 red peppers, deseeded and cut into 3cm cubes
200g (7oz) tin chopped tomatoes
400ml (10fl.oz) vegetable stock
250g (9oz) couscous
410g (14oz) can chickpeas, drained and rinsed
60g (2oz) black olives, pitted
A little low-sodium salt and freshly ground black pepper

1. Heat the olive oil in a large nonstick pan. Add the onions and aubergine and cook gently for 10 minutes, stirring occasionally. Add the spices, stir and continue cooking for a few moments. Dice the whole lemon, including the skin. Add to the aubergine with the courgettes and red peppers.

2. Add the tomatoes and pour in the stock. Stir and bring to the boil. Cover, then simmer for 15 minutes or until the vegetables are tender.

3. While the tagine is cooking, put the couscous in a bowl and add boiling water until just covered. Leave for 15 minutes, drain, then transfer back to the bowl. Fluff with a fork and keep warm.

4. Add the chickpeas, olives and seasoning. Bring back to the boil, then serve with the couscous.

Lentil and red pepper dahl

Makes 4 servings

2 onions, chopped
1 large red pepper, deseeded and chopped

2tbsp (30ml) rapeseed oil
2 garlic cloves, crushed
1tsp (5ml) ground cumin
2tsp (10ml) ground coriander
1tsp (5ml) turmeric
175g (6oz) red lentils
750ml (1¼ pints) vegetable stock
1tbsp (15ml) lemon juice
A little low-sodium salt
A small handful of fresh coriander, finely chopped

1. Heat the oil in a heavy-based pan and sauté the onions and red pepper for 5 minutes. Add the garlic and spices and continue cooking for 1 minute while stirring continuously.
2. Add the lentils and stock. Bring to the boil. Cover and simmer for about 20 minutes.
3. Add the lemon juice and low-sodium salt. Finally, stir in the fresh coriander. Serve topped with a spoonful of natural yoghurt.

Sweet-and-sour chicken with mango

Makes 4 servings

For the sweet-and-sour sauce:
4tbsp water
2tbsp each dry sherry, sesame oil and white-wine vinegar
1tbsp light soy sauce
2tsp honey
For the chicken:
1 large mango

2tbsp sunflower oil
4 chicken breast fillets, cut into 1cm pieces
2 onions, sliced
250g (9oz) broccoli, divided into small florets
1tsp grated fresh ginger

1. For the sauce, combine the water, sherry, sesame oil, vinegar, soy
    sauce and honey.
2. Slice through the mango either side of the stone. Peel, then cut
    the flesh into cubes.
3. Heat half the sunflower oil in a wok or large frying pan, add
    the chicken and quickly brown on all sides for 2 to 3 minutes.
    Transfer to a warm plate.
4. Heat the remaining oil, add the onions and cook for 1 or 2
    minutes until softened. Add the broccoli and ginger followed by
    the sauce and the mango.
5. Bring to the boil and then simmer gently for 3 minutes. Return
    the chicken to the wok and continue to cook for a further 2 to 3
    minutes until thoroughly cooked. Serve with basmati rice.

Fish with spicy chickpeas

Makes 4 servings

1 lemon, zest and juice
3tbsp olive oil
4×140g (5oz) white-fish fillets (e.g. halibut, haddock, monkfish or
    Icelandic cod), skinned
1 onion, sliced into thin wedges
1 red pepper, sliced

250g (9oz) packet fresh spinach, stems trimmed
½–1tsp dried chilli flakes
410g (14oz) canned chickpeas, rinsed and drained
A small handful of fresh coriander, chopped

1. To cook the fish: Preheat the grill. Mix the lemon zest with 1tbsp of the olive oil. Line a roasting tin with foil, oil lightly and add the fish. Brush the fish with the lemon oil. Season and grill for 8 to 10 minutes until cooked (no need to turn it).

2. Meanwhile, heat the rest of the oil and cook the onion and pepper over a moderate heat until translucent. Add the spinach and cook for a minute until wilted. Stir in the chilli flakes. Tip in the chickpeas and 1tbsp of lemon juice, heat through and season. Spoon the chickpea mixture onto hot plates and serve the fish on top. Scatter over the coriander and drizzle with a little extra oil or lemon juice.

Tarragon chicken breasts on lentils and mushrooms

Makes 4 servings

1tbsp olive oil
4 leeks, sliced
150ml (5fl.oz) white wine
8 tarragon sprigs
4×150g (5oz) skinless chicken breasts, cut lengthways into 4 pieces
Freshly ground black pepper
250g (9oz) pack ready-cooked puy lentils (or tinned)

125g (4oz) button mushrooms
125g (4oz) fresh tomatoes, halved or quartered

1. Heat the oil in a large heavy-bottomed pan, add the leeks and cook over a low heat for 10 minutes. Add the wine and boil until almost reduced.
2. Scatter the tarragon sprigs over the leeks and lay the chicken pieces on top. Season with the black pepper. Cover the pan and simmer for 15 to 18 minutes until the chicken is cooked.
3. Meanwhile, mix the lentils, mushrooms and fresh tomatoes in a saucepan. Bring to the boil, reduce the heat then simmer for 10 minutes until slightly thickened.
4. Divide the lentil mixture onto 4 plates, then spoon the cooked chicken on top.

Roast vegetable and bean lasagne

Makes 8 servings

1 large butternut squash, peeled and diced
1 red pepper, cut into strips
1 yellow pepper, cut into strips
2 courgettes, trimmed and thickly sliced
2 red onions, cut into wedges
½ an aubergine, cut into 2cm cubes
125g (4oz) cherry tomatoes
A few sprigs of rosemary
1 garlic clove, crushed
4tbsp (60ml) extra-virgin olive oil
400g tin chopped tomatoes
400g tomato pasta sauce

400g tin mixed beans, drained and rinsed

600ml (1 pint) cheese sauce

175g (6oz) lasagne sheets (not pre-cooked)

1. Preheat the oven to 200°C/400°F/Gas mark 6.
2. Place all the vegetables in a large roasting tin. Place the rosemary sprigs between the vegetables and scatter over the crushed garlic. Drizzle over the olive oil and toss lightly so that the vegetables are well coated in the oil.
3. Roast in the oven for about 30 minutes until the vegetables are slightly charred on the outside and tender in the middle.
4. Remove the vegetables from the oven and add the tinned tomatoes, pasta sauce and drained beans, then stir to combine.
5. Place a layer of lasagne sheets in a lightly oiled baking dish. Cover with one third of the vegetable mixture then one third of the cheese sauce. Continue with the layers, finishing with the cheese sauce.
6. Bake at 200°C/400°F/Gas mark 6 for 40 to 45 minutes.

Puy lentils with Mediterranean vegetables

Makes 4 servings

2tbsp olive oil

1 medium red pepper, diced

1 medium yellow pepper, diced

1 small red onion

1 medium courgette, thinly sliced

250g (9oz) pack ready-cooked puy lentils (or tinned)

Zest and juice of 1 lime

Freshly ground black pepper
60g (2oz) feta cheese, diced

1. Heat the olive oil in a nonstick pan. Add the peppers and onion and sauté over a gentle heat for 2 minutes. Add the courgettes and cook for a further minute. Add 2tbsp of water, cover the pan and cook for a further 5 minutes until the vegetables are just tender.
2. Add the lentils, lime zest and juice and stir well. Season with black pepper, add the feta cheese and mix together.
3. Serve with a leafy salad and baked potatoes.

Chicken soup

Makes 4 servings

> 2tbsp olive oil
> 2 onions, finely sliced
> 2 potatoes, peeled and diced
> 2 stalks celery, thinly sliced
> 1 carrots, thinly sliced
> 2 skinless chicken breasts, diced
> 1 litre (1¾ pints) chicken stock
> 400g (13oz) tin chickpeas, drained and rinsed
> 1 bay leaf
> 1tbsp chopped chives or parsley

1. Heat the olive oil in a large heavy-based saucepan. Add the onion, potatoes, celery, carrots and diced chicken. Cook gently for about 5 minutes or until the vegetables have softened.
2. Pour in the stock, add the chickpeas and bay leaf and bring to

the boil. Simmer, partially covered, for a further 15 to 20 minutes until the vegetables are tender.

3. Stir in the fresh herbs and serve.

Leek and potato soup

Makes 4 servings

> 1 litre (1¾ pints) vegetable stock
> 3 medium potatoes, scrubbed and roughly chopped
> 3 large leeks, sliced
> 1 large carrot, sliced
> A little low-sodium salt and freshly ground black pepper
> A small handful of chopped fresh parsley

1. Place the vegetable stock, potatoes, leeks and carrots in a large saucepan. Bring to the boil, lower the heat, cover and simmer for about 20 minutes until the vegetables are tender.
2. Remove from the heat and liquidise until smooth using a blender, food processor or a hand blender.
3. Return to the saucepan to heat through. Season the soup with the low-sodium salt and freshly ground black pepper. Stir in the fresh parsley.

Dessert Recipes

Apple sorbet

> 1 litre (1¾ pints) freshly pressed apple juice
> A little icing sugar
> Lemon juice

1. Whisk a little icing sugar and lemon juice into your apple juice to get the right balance of sweetness and acid.
2. Then either churn in an ice-cream maker or pour into plastic dishes to a depth of no more than 2cm (¾ inch). If you're using plastic dishes, then remove them from the freezer when the mixture is just frozen (but not rock hard) and scratch up into a soft sorbet using a fork.
3. Either serve straightaway or pack into tubs and freeze. Defrost for 30 to 60 minutes at room temperature before serving.

Raspberry and passion fruit fool

Makes 4 servings

1 small passion fruit
200g (7oz) raspberries
1 tbsp lemon juice
2 tbsp golden caster sugar
2 large egg whites
300ml (½ pint) low-fat Greek-style yoghurt

1. Halve the passion fruit and scoop the pulp into a medium-sized bowl. Add the raspberries and lemon juice with 1 tbsp of the caster sugar. Stir lightly with a wooden spoon, crushing the fruit just enough to release some of their juices, but still keeping the raspberries whole. Set aside for 10 minutes.
2. Meanwhile, whisk the egg whites until stiff peaks form. Gradually whisk in the remaining 1 tbsp of sugar until thick and glossy.
3. Combine the yoghurt and fruit. Then, using a metal spoon, fold in

the egg whites. Divide between 4 serving glasses and chill until firm, for up to 2 hours.

Spiced fruit skewers

Makes 4 servings

50g (2oz) clear honey

1 tbsp lemon juice

Juice of 1 orange

8 cardamom pods, lightly crushed

1 cinnamon stick, halved

8 Medjool dates, pitted

8 apricots, halved and stoned

4 plums, stoned and halved

1. Place the honey, lemon juice, orange juice, cardamom pods and cinnamon stick in a shallow dish. Add the dates, apricots and plums. Marinate for at least 30 minutes.

2. Drain the fruits, reserving the honey syrup, and thread onto 4 long wooden skewers. Cook under a preheated grill (or over a prepared barbecue) for 10 to 15 minutes, or until beginning to colour.

Exotic fruit salad

Makes 4 servings

2 tbsp clear honey

100ml (3fl.oz) water

Zest of 1 lime

20g pack fresh mint leaves
1 pineapple, skin removed, quartered and cored
3 kiwi fruit, peeled and cut into chunks
1 mango, peeled and sliced

1. Place the honey, water and lime zest and half the mint in a jug. Allow to infuse for 1 hour, then strain.
2. Cut the pineapple into small wedges and toss gently in a large bowl with the kiwi fruit and mango pieces. Pour the cooled syrup over and combine well.
3. Divide the fruit between 4 bowls, decorate with the remaining mint and serve with natural yoghurt.

Roasted peaches and plums with yoghurt

Makes 4 servings

4 ripe peaches
4 ripe plums
1 cinnamon stick, broken in half
Zest and juice of 2 oranges
2tbsp clear honey
400g (14oz) natural yoghurt

1. Preheat the oven to 200°C/400°F/Gas mark 6. Halve and stone the peaches and plums and arrange, cut-side up, in a shallow dish large enough to hold them all in one layer.
2. Put the cinnamon stick, orange zest and juice and honey in a small pan. Heat gently until the honey has melted. Pour evenly over the fruit. Roast in the oven for 25 to 30 minutes, basting halfway though the cooking time, until the fruit is tender.

3. Cool for 10 minutes then divide between serving plates. Place a dessertspoonful of yoghurt into the cavity of each fruit and drizzle some of the honey syrup over. Serve the rest of the yoghurt separately.

Oaty apple crumble

Makes 4 servings

700g (1½lb) cooking apples, peeled and sliced
85g (3oz) clear honey
½tsp cinnamon
4tbsp (60ml) water
For the topping:
125g (4oz) plain flour
85g (3oz) olive oil margarine
50g (2oz) oats
75g (2½oz) brown sugar

1. Preheat the oven to 190°C/375°C/Gas mark 5.
2. Place the apples, honey and cinnamon in a deep baking dish. Combine well and pour the water over.
3. For the crumble topping, put the flour in a bowl and rub in the margarine until the mixture resembles coarse breadcrumbs. Mix in the oats and sugar. Alternatively, mix in a food mixer or processor.
4. Sprinkle the crumble mixture over the fruit. Bake for 20 to 25 minutes until the topping is golden and the fruit is tender.

Poached pears with cinnamon

Makes 4 servings

  250ml (8fl.oz) red wine

  2tbsp light-brown sugar

  2 cinnamon sticks

  5 whole cloves

  4 pears, peeled and halved

  Plain bio-yoghurt to serve

1. Place the wine, sugar and spices in a saucepan just large
    enough to fit the pears. Bring slowly to the boil, stirring
    occasionally until the sugar has dissolved.

2. Add the pears and simmer gently for 20 minutes until they are
    tender.

3. Remove the pears with a slotted spoon and set aside. Turn
    the heat up and boil the cooking liquor until it reduces by half.
    Remove the spices. Serve the pears with their liquor and
    yoghurt.

Baked apples with blackberries

Makes 4 servings

  4 Bramley cooking apples

  4tbsp clear honey

  ½tsp ground cinnamon

  Zest of 1 orange

  250g (9oz) blackberries

  1tbsp (15ml) pecans, chopped

1. Preheat the oven to 190°C/375°F/Gas mark 5.
2. Remove the core from the apples. Using a sharp knife, lightly score the skin around the middle, just enough to pierce the skin.
3. Stand the apples in a shallow baking dish large enough to fit all four snugly side by side. In a small bowl, combine the honey, cinnamon and orange zest. Spoon into the cavities of the apples. Pour 2tbsp of water into the dish, cover loosely with foil then bake for 40 minutes, spooning the cooking juices over occasionally.
4. Spoon the blackberries over and around the apples, scatter over the pecans then return to the oven for 10 minutes. Serve warm.

Tropical fruit salad with lime fromage frais

Makes 4 servings

1 papaya
1 mango
½ a fresh pineapple
Zest of 1 lime
4tbsp plain fromage frais

1. Cut the papaya flesh into cubes. Slice through the mango either side of the stone. Peel, then cut the flesh into cubes. Cut the pineapple into 4×1cm (½-inch) rounds then cut each round into quarters. Place the fruit in a large bowl.
2. Mix the lime zest with the fromage frais. Serve the fruit with the lime fromage frais.

Melon and raspberries

Makes 4 servings

½ a cantaloupe melon
¼ of a watermelon
Zest and juice of 1 orange
150g (5oz) raspberries
Orange liqueur (optional)

1. Scoop out the seeds from the cantaloupe melon, cut into slices, peel and slice into chunks. Cut the watermelon into chunks, discarding skin and any seeds.
2. Place the melon pieces in a large bowl; add the orange zest and juice, and raspberries. Combine together. Add a splash of orange liqueur, if you wish, then serve with low-fat yoghurt.

Index